Recent Research on Balance Disorders

Edited by Esor Balkan

Published in London, United Kingdom

Recent Research on Balance Disorders
http://dx.doi.org/10.5772/intechopen.105655
Edited by Esor Balkan

Contributors
Renu Rajguru, Maria Cristina Alves Corazza, Luíza Alves Corazza, Júlia Alves Corazza, Paul S. Sung, Dongchul Lee, Neil S. Longridge, Esor Balkan

First published in London, United Kingdom, 2023 by IntechOpen
IntechOpen is the global imprint of INTECHOPEN LIMITED, registered in England and Wales, registration number: 11086078, 5 Princes Gate Court, London, SW7 2QJ, United Kingdom

British Library Cataloguing-in-Publication Data
A catalogue record for this book is available from the British Library

Additional hard and PDF copies can be obtained from orders@intechopen.com

Recent Research on Balance Disorders
Edited by Esor Balkan
p. cm.
Print ISBN 978-1-83768-766-4
Online ISBN 978-1-83768-767-1
eBook (PDF) ISBN 978-1-83768-768-8

Meet the editor

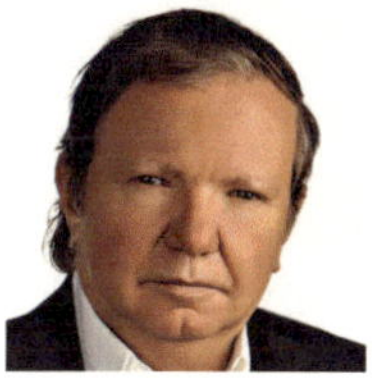

Prof. Dr. Esor Balkan is the manager of vertigo clinics in Istanbul and Antalya, Turkey. He has researched balance disorders for about 15 years. Dr. Balkan is a member of the ENT Society and has published numerous journal articles and book chapters.

Contents

Preface

Balance disorders significantly affect the quality of life. Due to the complexity of balance physiology, the diagnosis and treatment of balance disorders require meticulous research. Even today, the functioning of the peripheral and central organs that make up the balance system is not clearly known.

With the development of technology, a new set of electrophysiological tests have been developed and found to help with balance disorders. In addition, these tests have illuminated many aspects of the balance system that were previously hidden in the dark. However, this information is still not sufficient and new scientific research is required.

Since the balance system is not dependent on a single organ, it requires multidisciplinary research. First, it is essential to know how to approach a patient who presents with a complaint of balance disorder and vertigo. For this, it is necessary to know the anatomy and physiology of the balance organs. In addition, it is necessary to know the laboratory tools that may be necessary for diagnosis.

This book summarizes how we should approach patients with balance disorder and presents valuable studies in the field. It is a useful resource for healthcare professionals as well as training practitioners working in polyclinics and emergency departments.

Esor Balkan
Private ENT and VERTIGO Clinic Antalya,
Antalya, Turkey

Section 1

Introduction

Chapter 1

Introductory Chapter: Balance Disorders

Esor Balkan

1. Introduction

We owe our balance to our vestibular system to work correctly and in harmony with other systems in our body. Although the balance system is complex, we can maintain our balance due to the smooth and harmonious operation of the factors that build up this system. Knowing the anatomical and physiological factors that make up these systems is essential for the treatment of balance system disorders. Researches are still needed for the subject of balance disorders.

These systems are the following:

1. Vestibular systems

    a. Peripheral vestibular system

    b. Central vestibular system

2. Proprioceptive system

3. Visual system.

    a. The peripheral system anatomically starts from the cupulas of horizontal, superior, and posterior semicircular canals and from the utriculus and the sacculus in the vestibule.

       The system continues with the vestibular nerve and ends at the four vestibular nuclei in the brainstem.

    b. The central vestibular system consists of the connections of these four nuclei with the cerebellum, spinal cord, extraocular eye muscles, and the vestibular cortex in the brain.

When the information about the body's position coming from the peripheral vestibular system, proprioceptive system, and the eyes reaches the central vestibular system, as inputs in the central system, these sensory stimuli are processed. The central vestibular system then creates the motor impulses to the muscles necessary to keep the body in balance (**Figure 1**) [1].

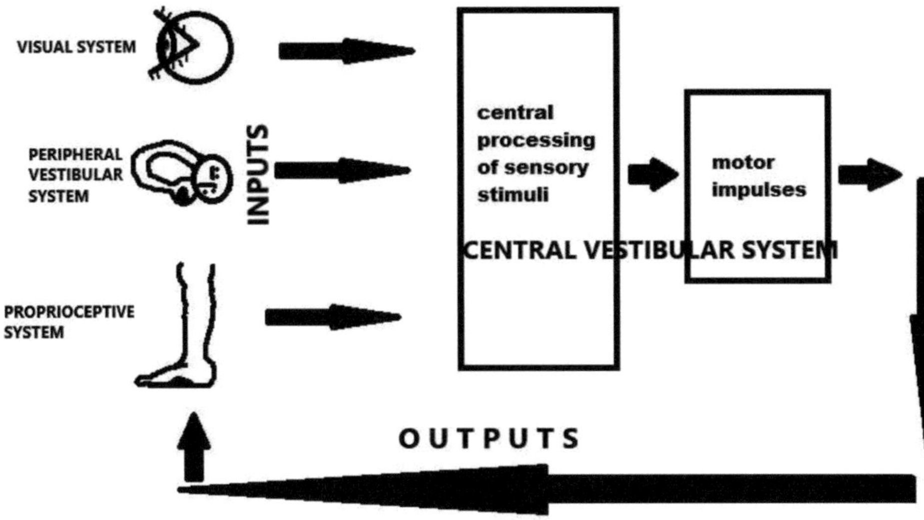

Figure 1.
Balance system.

Any pathology of both peripheral and central vestibular systems may cause deterioration of our balance. This disorder is described by patients as vertigo, dizziness, disequilibrium, unsteadiness, and lightheadedness [2].

Other than peripheral and central vestibular systems, the cardiovascular system, endocrine system, eye, psychic stability, and even some orthopedic disorders can cause balance disorders. For these reasons, it is necessary to think of a broad-spectrum in patients presenting with the complaints of balance disorders as described above and to approach these patients in a multidisciplinary manner. During a multidisciplinary approach, while the group of common diseases comes to mind first, it should be kept in mind that there may be more than one factor that may disturb the balance in a patient [3]. Asking the patient the style of the balance disorder, whether there are any accompanying complaints such as headaches, hearing loss, tinnitus, darkening, that is, a detailed story of the patient, will provide almost half of our diagnosis [4]. After that, we can make a definitive diagnosis by evaluating the laboratory tests together with the physical examinations that we make. To diagnose balance disorders, we have to perform a series of examinations and tests, such as neurological examinations, balance tests (VNG, Caloric tests, Posturographic tests, etc.), and imaging studies such as MRI, CT scan [5].

In this book, we wanted to gather all these thoughts together, search for more new research, and show how to approach a patient with a balance disorder.

We hope to help our physicians who are dealing with balance disorders.

Author details

Esor Balkan
Private ENT and VERTIGO Clinic Antalya, Turkey

*Address all correspondence to: esorbalkan@gmail.com

References

[1] Luxon LM. Overview of Balance. Chapter 19. Scott Browns otolaryngology. In: Kerr AG, editor. Adult Audiology. 6th. ed. Vol. 2. London: Hodder Education; 1997. pp. 1-10

[2] Brandt T. Vertigo. It's Multisensory Syndromes. London: Springer Verlag; 1990

[3] Mahoney CF, Luxon LM. Causes of balance disorders. Chapter 20. In: Kerr AG, editor. Scott Brown's Otolaryngology. 6th ed. Vol. 2. Adult Audiology. London: Hodder Education; 1997. pp. 1-57

[4] Solomon D. Practical issues in the management of the dizzy and balance disorder patient. In: Otolaryngol. Clinic. North Am. New York: WB Saunders; 2000. pp. 33-33

[5] Derebery MJ. Otolaryngology fort the internist. The diagnosis and treatment of dizziness. The Medical Clinics of North America. 1999;**83**:163-176

Section 2

Initial Approach to Balance Disorders

Chapter 2

Initial Approach to Patients with Balance Disorders

Esor Balkan

Abstract

Balance disorders can be due to many different reasons. Some possible causes are: Inner ear problems: Located in the inner ear, the vestibular system controls the balance of the body. Factors such as infections, traumas or aging in the inner ear can affect the vestibular system and cause imbalances. Brain damage: Damage to the brain, especially damage to areas responsible for balance control, such as the brain stem, cerebral cortex, and cerebellum, can cause imbalances. Nervous system problems: Nervous system problems can cause imbalances by causing problems in communicating with your body's sensory information and motor functions. Medication side effects: Some medications can cause symptoms such as dizziness or unsteadiness as a side effect. Eye disorders: Visual disturbances, especially problems with coordination between the eyes or damage to the retina, can cause imbalances. Low blood pressure: Low blood pressure can also cause imbalance, especially when you get up suddenly or go to high altitudes. Stress and anxiety: Stress and anxiety can cause symptoms such as dizziness and unsteadiness in some people.

Keywords: balance, vertigo, dizziness, initial approach, treatment

1. Introduction

Achieving balance depends on the harmonious functioning of the vestibular system, proprioceptive system, and visual systems. Disorders of the balance system can cause a wide range of symptoms, defined as vertigo, dizziness, and sudden falls of the patients.

Vertigo is not a disease name, it is a hallucination of the spinning of the patient himself or his surroundings, caused by an unusual stimulation of the vestibular system. These stimuli are either physiological or pathological. There are three systems that keep our balance [1].

2. Vestibular system

The vestibular system is the most important part of the human balance system. It consists of two parts:

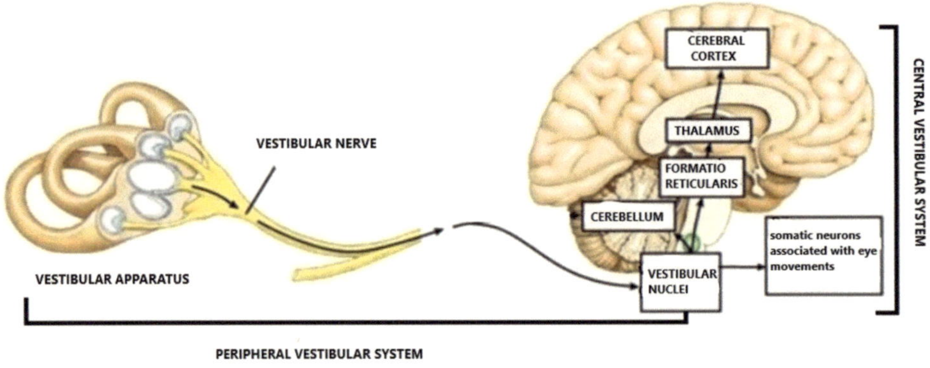

Figure 1.
Vestibular system.

a. Peripheral Vestibular System: Systems starting from the vestibular apparatus (semicircular canals, utriculus, and sacculus) till to the vestibular nuclei in the brain stem.

b. Central Vestibular System: It consists of parts starting from the brain stem to the cerebellum, formatio reticularis, thalamus, and vestibular cortex (**Figure 1**).

When there is a problem in one of these systems, the cortex perceives this disorder as a movement and rotation of the body. Vertigo is the result of this misperception.

3. Proprioceptive system

They are the pathways that transmit position and movement signals from the joints and muscles to the brain.

4. Visual system

It is an important part of the balance system that informs the position of our head to the central vestibular system.

In addition, the cardiovascular and hematological systems are necessary for the correct functioning of the whole vestibular system.

Vertigo is the movement hallucination that develops with the unusual stimulation of these systems, either without a disease (physiological) or due to a disease (pathological).

A person becomes dizzy when he suddenly stops after turning around quickly several times. The event here is the unusual stimulation of the semicircular canals in the inner ear. Dizziness occurs in people who are not accustomed to looking down from extreme heights. These are examples of physiological vertigo. Pathological vertigos, on the other hand, are vertigos due to diseases that affect the systems that maintain our balance. Therefore, pathological vertigo requires a multidisciplinary approach [2].

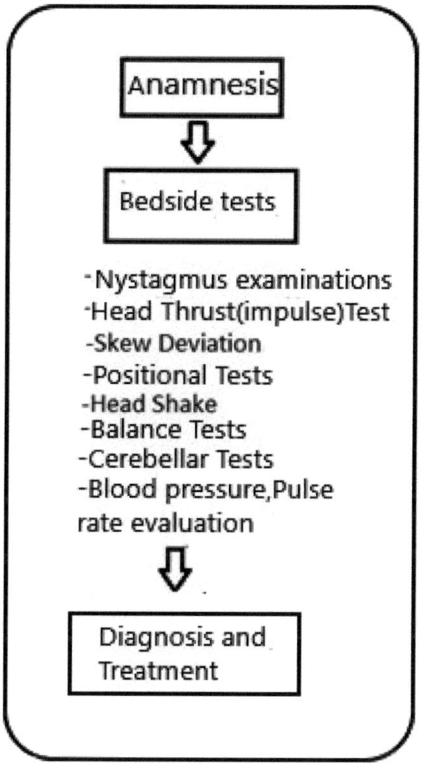

Figure 2.
Algorithm of evaluation of patients with vertigo.

When the patient comes to the doctor, he says "I feel dizzy" or "I have vertigo". In such a case, our approach to the patient should be with an algorithm (**Figure 2**).

The first step of the algorithm should be the inquiry, that is, ANAMNESIS.

Vertigo-causing diseases are usually either specific or have common characteristics with other diseases. For this reason, inquiries should not be made randomly, but with questions that will include the characters of those diseases. The most important way to affect the treatment of a patient with vertigo is correct anamnesis. When choosing these questions, it is necessary to know the diseases that cause vertigo.

These questions will make it easier to reach the diagnosis

a. Asking about the form and duration of complaints. It is a great guide in the differentiation of peripheral, central, cardiovascular, and psychic causes.

b. Factors triggering complaints. They are guiding questions in the differentiation of common causes of vertigo, especially vestibular migraines, BPPV.

c. Additional events accompanying the complaints. These are important questions, especially for the definition of Meniere's disease, migraine, and some other central or psychic vertigos

d. Duration and continuity of the complaints. Asking whether the vertigo is in the form of attacks, whether it is continuous and if it is in attacks, the duration of the vertigo are questions that make it easier to distinguish peripheral diseases from central pathologies.

e. Self and family history. Asking whether the patient has other systemic diseases and family history may also help in the diagnosis.

5. Anamnesis questions

5.1 Forms of complaints

- ☐ **Turning sensation of one's self or around** – perıpheric or central pathology?
- ☐ **Feeling of fainting** – usually neuro cardiogenic, orthostatic pathology?
- ☐ **Imbalance** – usually central, proprioceptive or bilateral peripheral pathologies?
- ☐ **Sway** – possible central pathology?
- ☐ **Tendency to fall to one side** – possible unilateral peripheral pathologies?
- ☐ **Floating sensation** – possible central, visual, psycho-somatic pathologies?
- ☐ **Feeling like walking in space** – medications, possible metabolic disorders?
- ☐ **Vision darkening** – possible vasovagal attacks, cardiogenic, orthostatic dysregulations?
- ☐ **Loss of consiousness** – possible epilepsy.
- ☐ or **Other**............

5.2 Complaint initiating stimuli

- ☐ **Rapid head movement** – peripheral pathology?
- ☐ **Head and body position changes** – BPPV?
- ☐ **Walking in a dark room** – proprioceptive, central pathologies?
- ☐ **Loud noises** – migraine, superior SSC dehiscence pathologies? Meniere's disease (Tullio phenomenon)
- ☐ **Blowing nose** – labyrinthine fistula, SSSC dehiscence?
- ☐ **Some foods** – migraine?
- ☐ **Stress** – migraine, psychosomatic?
- ☐ **Standing up swiftly** – orthostatic dysregulation?
- ☐ **Airplane or car ride** – migraine, motion sickness?
- ☐ **In malls or supermarkets** – migraine?, PPPD (persistent postural perceptual dizziness)?.
- ☐ **Menstrueal periods** – migraine?
- ☐ **Exercise** – migraine or cardiac diseases?
- ☐ **Head trauma** – migraine or central pathologies?
- ☐ or **Other**............

5.3 Accompanying complaints

☐ **Hearing loss – unilateral** Meniere, Labyrinthitis, tumor?
- Bilateral ototoxic medicaments, central?
☐ **Tinnitus – Meniere**, Tumor?
☐ **Fullness in the ear – Meniere**?
☐ **Fear, depression, crying, panic etc.** – psychiatric, somatoform?
☐ **Double or blurred vision** – vertebrobasillar disease, migraine, visual?
☐ **Photophobia** – migraine?
☐ **Feeling of emptiness in the head presyncope** – vasovagal?
☐ **Headache** – migraine, hypertension?
☐ **Disorders in any organ (sight, smell, taste etc..)** – epilepsy, migraine?
☐ or **Other**...........
☐ **Hearing in echoes** – acoustic **neuroma**, Meniere?
☐ **Impairement in walking – central** or Proprioceptive pathology?
☐ **Nausea-vomiting – peripheral** or central pathology?

5.4 Duration of complaints

☐ **Continuous**
V. Neuritis, Migraine?
☐ **by İctal periods**
Epilepsy?
☐ **2–3 sec**. Orthostatic,?
Psychogenic?
☐ **Minutes**
Migraine, Meniere's Disease?
☐ **Hours** Meniere's Disease, Migraine Stroke?
☐ **Days** V. Neuritis,
Meniere's Disease
☐ **Months.**
Cardiogenic, Central Nervous system tumors?

Familial or past illnesses: ....?
To rank these diseases according to their incidence rates [3]:

1. The most common peripheral vestibular system diseases: benign paroxysmal positional vertigo (BPPV), vestibular neuronitis, Meniere, labyrinthitis.

2. The most common central vestibular system diseases: vestibular migraine, cerebrovascular diseases.

3. The most common deep sensory system diseases: spinal dorsal root diseases such as Tabes dorsalis, disk pathologies.

4. Eye diseases, Sudden visual disturbances.

In addition to the symptom of vertigo, some patients may complain of feelings such as imbalance, shaking, being pushed, a feeling of emptiness in the head, and dizziness, and may describe these complaints as dizziness. The Anglo-Saxons named such complaints DIZZINESS. In order to distinguish such complaints from true vertigo, the doctor should ask what the vertigo complaint is like in the anamnesis. First of all, the questions should be selected according to the symptoms of these diseases. Shows the questions that can lead to the diagnosis.

6. Bedside tests

These are the examinations to be done in the first place.

a. Nystagmus examination

b. Head thrust test (head impulse test)

c. Eye cover test for skew deviation

d. Positional tests

e. Head shake test

f. Balance tests (Romberg and Fukuda)

g. Cerebellar examinations (dysdiacokinesia, knee-heel test)

h. Blood pressure measurement and pulse assessment.

i. Nystagmus examination: Nystagmus is the involuntary movements of the eyeballs. In order to maintain our balance in head and body movements, external object images must fall into the fovea in accordance with the movements. This is provided by the vestibulo-ocular reflex (VOR). Here, nystagmus develops as a result of an imbalance in this vestibulo-ocular reflex. It is very diverse.

Nystagmus are classified according to their i. their direction, ii. their phases, and iii. Their severity.

Nystagmus are observed as horizontal, vertical, or rotatory according to their direction [4].

They are biphasic (fast and slow phase) or monophasic (single phase).

They are divided into three degrees according to their severity:

First-degree nystagmus: nystagmus that occurs when looking at the lesion side. Second-degree nystagmus is seen even when the patient is looking ahead. Third degree nystagmus is the nystagmus flashing toward the sick side even when looking on the healthy side (**Figure 3**).

These nystagmuses are either spontaneous, gaze (looking to one side), or occur as a result of a provocation. These provocations are revealed either by positional or head shake movements.

For nystagmus examination, the patient is made to look across, right, left, up, and down. It is determined whether there is nystagmus or no. If present, it is a sign of

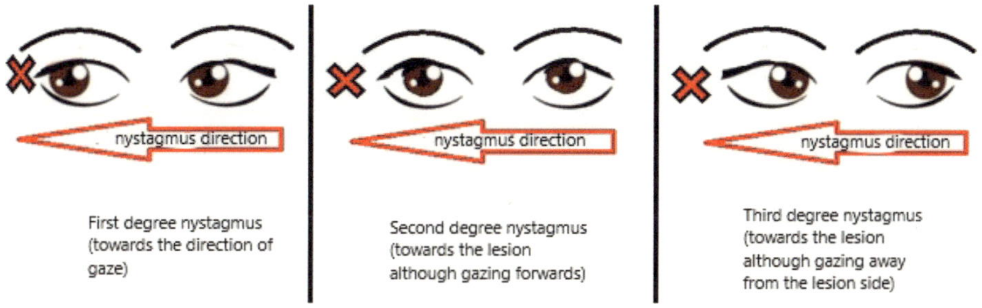

Figure 3.
Degrees of nystagmus.

either peripheral or central pathology. Nystagmus of peripheral diseases and nystagmus of central diseases are often different:

6.1 Peripheral nystagmus

1 – Horizontal or torsional. 2 – Direction is unilateral, and it does not change with the direction of gaze. 3 – Visual fixation suppresses nystagmus. 4 – It gets better within days. 5 – Dizziness is evident. 6 – Tinnitus may accompany. 7 – There are no additional brain stem and cerebellar signs.

6.2 Central nystagmus

1 – It has pure vertical, pure torsional, pure horizontal, or mixed appearance. 2 – Its direction changes with the gaze direction or it can be unilateral also. 3 – Visual fixation does not suppress nystagmus. 6 – It does not improve within days. 7 – Dizziness may not be evident. 8 – It is usually not accompanied by tinnitus. 9 – Brain stem findings and cerebellar findings may be present.

a. Head thrust (impulse) test: in this test, vestibulo ocular reflex (VOR) is examined. The patient is told to look fixedly at the doctor's nose, and the head is suddenly turned to one side. Normally, the eyes are fixed on the target even if the head is turned to one side. If it is observed that when the head is pushed to the lesion side, the eyes are directed to that side and then return to the target with a saccadic movement, and this is usually a sign of peripheral vestibulopathy (**Figure 4**).

b. In the skew deviatıon test, when the covered eye is uncovered suddenly, it is checked whether the eye makes a vertical movement or not. If there is such a movement, it is said that there is skew deviation. This is a sign of central pathology (**Figure 5**).

c. Positional tests: nystagmus during a positional test is the most common indicator of benign paroxysmal positional vertigo (BPPV) [3]. They may also give positive findings in some rare central or cervical events. Dix-Hallpike (**Figure 6**) and Roll tests (**Figure 7**) are done.

d. Head shake test: it is helpful in understanding the sick side in peripheral vertigo. Head shakes left and right several times and is stopped, and nystagmus begins to beat toward the healthy side [7]

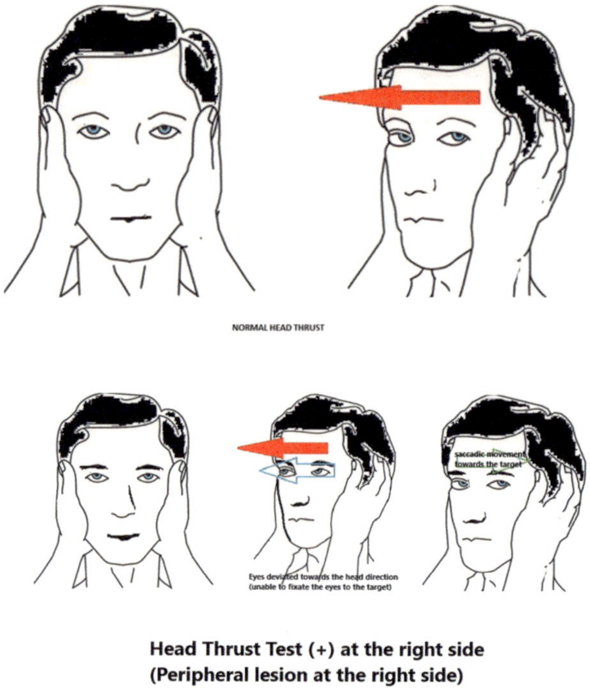

Figure 4.
Head thrust test positive on the right: The eyes are directed to the side where the head is turned, then back to the target [5, 6].

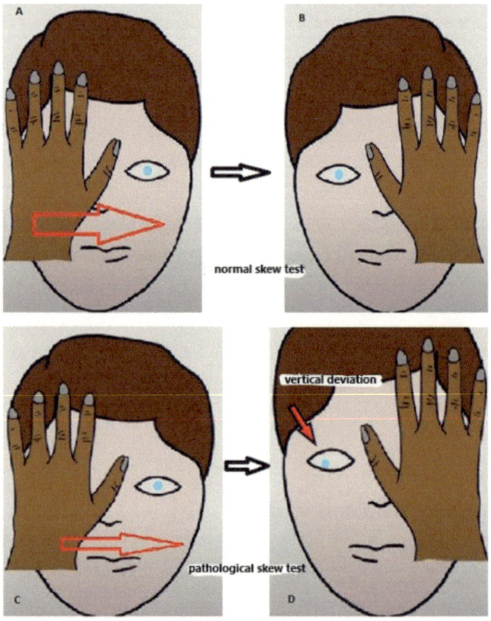

Figure 5.
Skew deviation test: Vertical movement of the eyeball is considered pathological when the eye is uncovered. (a, B normal skew test; C, D pathological skew test).

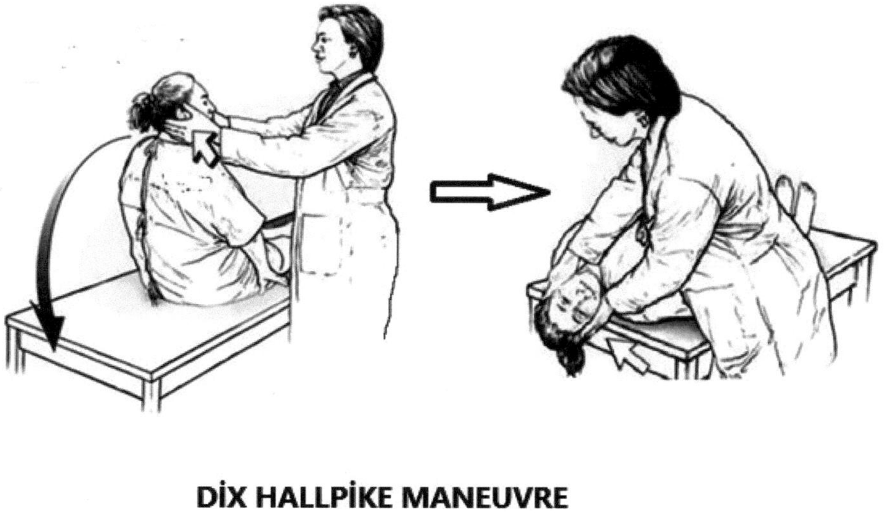

Figure 6.
Dix-Hallpike maneuver: Nystagmus in addition to severe vertigo indicates the presence of BPPV.

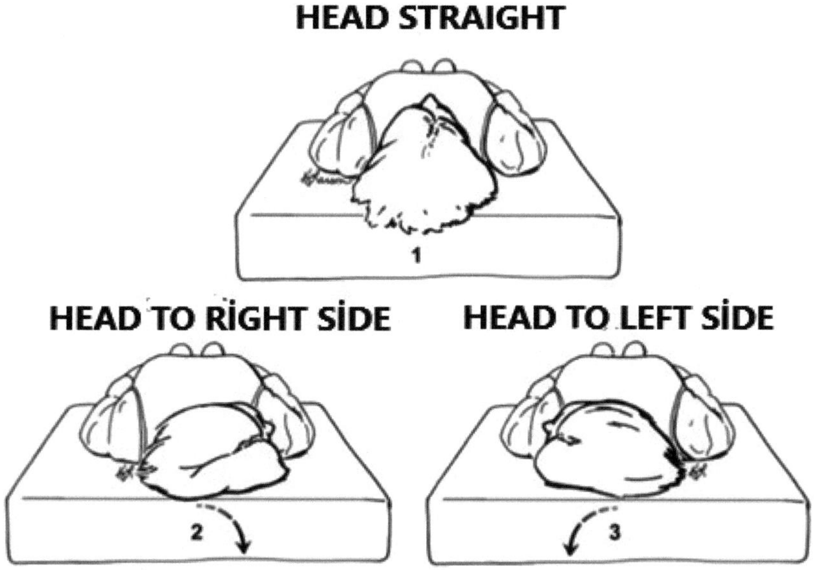

Figure 7.
Supine roll test: The patient is placed on his back and the head is turned to the right and left and the nystagmus is examined. If nystagmus occurs, it is in favor of BPPV.

e. Balance tests: Romberg and Fukuda.

In Romberg, the patient stands up and is told to put his legs together and close his eyes. If the patient's balance is disturbed when he closes his eyes, there is probably a neurological disorder in the deep sensory system. It requires neurology consultation.

In the Fukuda test [8], the patient is asked to step 50 times while standing, with his arms extended forward, with his eyes closed. It can be used to determine the side of the lesion in acute-stage vertigo. The patient deviates toward the lesion side.

g. Cerebellar tests: dysdiacokinesia (rotating one hand on the palm of the other hand) and knee-heel test (touching the heel of one foot to the knee of the other leg) are performed.

As a result of these preliminary examinations, it is tried to find out whether the vertigo is peripheral or central.

h. To rule out a cardiovascular pathology, blood pressure should be measured and pulse rate should be checked whether there is a rhythm disorder.

7. Most common peripheral vertigos

7.1 Benign paroxysmal positional vertigo (BPPV)

□ It is the most common type of peripheral vertigo.
□ Nystagmus is observed during acute transient vertigo attacks initiated by certain head positions and lasting seconds, minutes. Nystagmus decreases in repeated tests (tired nystagmus).
□ Calcium carbonate crystals called otoliths, which are attached to the utriculus and sacculus, break off and escape into the semicircular canals, creating this type of vertigo.

- They occur after factors such as head trauma, viral infection, after vestibular neuritis, degenerative disease, hypertension attack, migraine, or idiopathic.

- A sense of movement arises due to the reception of different signals from the contralateral vestibular system.

□ It is diagnosed by history and positional tests (Dix-Hallpike or Roll maneuvers).
□ Particle repositioning maneuvers are commonly used in treatment. These maneuvers vary according to the semicircular canal where the otoliths are located (e.g. Epley maneuver, Gufoni maneuvers, etc.). It is necessary to refer to an ENT specialist.

7.2 Meniere's disease

□ Pathogenesis: It begins as a result of insufficient absorption of endolymph and accumulation in the scala media of the inner ear (endolymphatic hydrops) [9].
□ Highest incidence (40–60 years),
□ Characterized by vertigo, hearing loss in one ear, tinnitus and a feeling of fullness in the ear, +/– falling attacks, nystagmus.
□ Vertigo (lasting about 20 minutes or 12 hours) disappears over time and the patient remains with only hearing loss.
□ In the early stages of the disease, hearing returns to normal during attack-free periods.

With the repetition of attacks, unilateral, low-frequency hearing loss becomes permanent.

□ Treatment

Bed rest in the acute period, IV antiemetics, antivertiginous drugs (dimenhydrinate, betahistine) (Serc). Besides the attack treatment, the therapeutic measures later in the attack-free period are very important Long-term follow-up with an ENT specialist is recommended.

7.3 Vestibular neuronitis

☐ Unknown etiology (it usually starts after an upper respiratory tract virus infections).
☐ Severe vertigo with nausea, vomiting, and inability to stand or walk.
☐ Acute symptoms may last 3 to 4 days (risk of dehydration from vomiting).
☐ The central compensation period can leave the patient unstable for months [10].
☐ Head thrust test is positive, and there is horızontal nystagmus beating toward the healthy side. Romberg is (+) toward the sick side. No hearing loss, no tinnitus, there is no feeling of fullness in the ear.

- Medications that suppress the vestibular system can be given in the first 48 hours to relieve vertigo, but they are not used continuously because they delay recovery. It is treated by an ENT specialist.

7.4 Labyrinthitis

This is an inflammation of the inner ear, mostly as a complication of middle ear infection.
☐ They develop as a result of an infection of the inner ear, mostly due to an infection of the middle ear, rarely after meningitis (labyrinth).
☐ Sudden onset of vertigo, nystagmus, nausea, vomiting, tınnıtus, and total hearing loss may be present. There is a history of ear discharge and pain.
☐ It is treated with IV antibiotics and sent to an ENT specialist for middle ear drainage and mastoidectomy.

8. The most common causes of central vertigo

Vestibular migraine [11], transient ischemic attack [12] (TIA) in the central nervous system (vertebrobasilar transient ischemic attack), cerebellar or brain stem strokes (stroke), less commonly cerebellopontine angle tumors, demyelination, or vertigo due to alcohol and drug toxicity.

The head thrust test is normal in central vertigo. While the nystagmus is generally vertical, they can also be horizontal or horizonto-rotatory. Nausea and vomiting are common in TIA and stroke. Peripheral findings such as tinnitus, hearing loss, and a feeling of fullness in the ear do not generally occur in central diseases, unless the stroke affects the anterior inferior cerebellar artery. Cerebellar tests are usually pathologic.

Patients with peripheral vertigo should be referred to ENT physicians, and if central vertigo is suspected, neurology or neurosurgery consultation should be requested while referring them to radiology for computerized tomography (CT) or magnetic resonance imaging (MRI).

In addition to vestibular system examinations, cardiovascular examinations should be performed in the patient who comes with the complaint of dizziness. While looking for the presence of hyper or hypotensıon, the presence of cardiac rhythm disorder should also be checked, and if a pathology is found, cardiology consultation should be requested.

9. Treatment

Treatment for balance disorders depends on the underlying cause. Some medications, physical therapy, or surgery may be needed. In some cases, vestibular migraine lifestyle changes such as avoiding certain foods and activities that trigger symptoms can be sufficient to manage the condition.

If there is an acute peripheral vertigo disease, antivertiginous and antiemetic drugs are applied as symptomatic treatment to relieve the patient. If there is no contraindication, preparations such as dimenhydrinate, piracetam, trimethobenzamidem, and betahistıne can be applied most frequently in emergency services.

Peripheral pathologies should be referred to ENT specialists, and central pathologies should be referred to neurology or neurosurgery.

Author details

Esor Balkan
Private ENT and VERTIGO Clinic Antalya, Turkey

*Address all correspondence to: esorbalkan@gmail.com

References

[1] Fuchs AF. The vestibular system. In: Patton HD, Fuchs AF, Hille B, Scher AM, Steiner R, editors. Textbook of Physiology. Vol. 1 Excitable Cells and Neurophysiology. Philadelphia: CWB Saunders; 1989. pp. 582-607

[2] Drahman DA, Hart CW. An approach to the dizzy patient. Neurology. 1972;**22**:325-334

[3] Dix MR, Hallpike CS. The pathology of symptomatology and diagnosis of certain common disorders of the vestibular system. Proceedings of the Royal Society of Medicine. 1952;**45**:341-354

[4] Leigh RJ, Rucker JC. Nystagmus and related ocular motility disorders. In: Miller NR, Newman NJ, editors. Walsh and Hoyt's. Clinical Neuro-Ophtalmology. Baltimore, MD: Lippincott. Williams and Wilkins; 2004

[5] Nelson JA, Virre E. The clinical differentiation of cerebellar infarction from common vertigo syndromes. Western. Journal of Emergency Medicine. Nov 2009;**10**(4):273-277

[6] Halmagyi GM, Curthoys IS. A clinical sign of canal paresis. Archives of Neurology. 1988;**45**:737-739

[7] Hain TC, Fetter M, Zee DS. Head shaking nystagmus in patients with unilateral peripheral vestibular lesions. American Journal of Laryngology & Otology. 1938;**53**:625-655

[8] The FT, Test S. Two phases of the labyrinthine reflex. Acta Oto-Laryngologica. 1958;**50**:95-108

[9] Hallpike CS, Cains H. Observations on the pathology of Meniere's syndrome. The Journal of Laryngology and Otology. 1938;**53**:625-655

[10] Dix MR, Hallpike CS. The pathology symptomatology and diagnosis of cCertain common Disordres of the vestibular system. Proceedings of the Royal Society of Medicine. 1952;**45**:341-354

[11] Kayan A, Hood J. Neuro-Otological manifestations of migraine. Brain. 1984;**107**:1123-1142

[12] Grad A, Baloh RW. Vertigo of vascular origin clinical and electronystagmographic features in 84cases. Archives of Neurology. 1989;**46**:281-284

Section 3

Research

Chapter 3

Critical Cochlea/Vestibular Interactions

Neil S. Longridge

Abstract

There is a close interaction of the gravity detecting balance organs, the maculae of the saccule and utricle of the inner ear, with the hearing system of the inner ear. The need for this is that although they detect the sensations specific to their own function there is interference with this function due to overlap of wavelengths used by both systems resulting in extraordinary stimulation of the other system for both hearing and balance.

Keywords: Cvemp, Ovemp, macula of the utricle, macula of the saccule, stapedius reflex, otoconia, superior semicircular canal dehiscence syndrome

1. Introduction

The precise way that the cochlea and vestibular system interact is not clearly understood. This chapter addresses this deficiency attempting to relate the cochlear and vestibular inter dependency, in such a way that it will effectively lead to research more clearly outlining this association, and hopefully result in more effective therapy for patients with both cochlear and vestibular diseases.

2. Vestibular evoked myogenic potentials. What are they?

Cervical vestibular evoked myogenic potentials (Cvemps) are a response to repetitive sound into the ipsilateral ear resulting in reduction of tonic activity of the tensed ipsilateral sternomastoid muscle. Ocular vestibular evoked myogenic potentials (Ovemp) responses are a contralateral sound or vibration excitatory reflex response and move the eyes in the direction of the stimulus. Ovemps are done with the eyes raised and tonic stimulation of the superior ophthalmic muscles is measured [1].

Why do these responses occur, what are they for. At first I assumed that the ear nearer the sound which hears a sound louder speeds a rapid head turn in the direction of the sound. Perhaps these Cvemp and Ovemp sound responses are the beginning of a fast reflex eye movement and head turn in the direction of a sound and in combination are protective by turning the head as rapidly as possible to look at what may be a potential threat.

If that is correct then why is there an Ovemp response with direct vibratory stimulation of the skull. A head blow is a normal life occurrence. The reflex produces a physiological stimulus causing the individual to look toward where the blow has arisen. Vibratory Ovemps are a response to a repetitive tap on the skull. Clearly, this is not a physiological stimulus produced by an external source [2]. Vibratory OVEMP's occur as a response to repetitive direct skull stimulation and are an externally measurable response to internally generated vibration from preplanned skull vibration, which occurs during chewing, speaking and other upper body internally generated vibrations. The externally recorded response is due to neural circuitry resulting in cochlea suppression of these internally generated sounds so that the threat of external potentially hazardous sound can be specifically differentiated from internal stimuli by the cochlea.

The stimulus used for sound Cvemp is a 95 dB, 500 Hz air conduction signal and for Ovemp induction in our laboratory is a 97 dB SPL,500 Hz air conduction signal [1].

These stimuli are considerably above any commonly occurring natural external sounds. Sounds louder than this do occur in nature, at waterfalls, for example, Niagara Falls also waves breaking at the seashore, with roaring animals, barking dogs and during thunder storms. In terms of an evolutionarily benefit, these sounds are so rare that it is unlikely that complex vestibular and cochlea responses of the sort described as causing vemp responses would have developed as a consequence of these rare occurrences. Also, Cvemps and Ovemps are done by having the patient take up an activity that is rarely done in normal life and requires an aphysiologically loud external sound stimulus. Persistent tonic sternomastoid contraction is not often undertaken. Head turn is usually a rapid response to a stimulus. Ovemp is done by having the eyes elevated 30 degrees. In life, this is done only briefly before the head is raised. The fact that unusual activities are needed to produce responses raises the question of what useful purpose they serve. Cvemps and Ovemps are extremely helpful to the clinician allowing detection of malfunction of the macula of the saccule and utricle respectively and in this they appear to be akin to the auditory brainstem responses [ABR] that are extremely helpful for the physician in perhaps suggesting the presence of an acoustic neuroma but do not as far as we know have a specific physiological function of their own.

Sound Ovemps at 500 Hertz the standard frequency used during this test are more difficult to record reliably than vibration Ovemps [2]. This is because the response to sound stimulation is only just above the level of electrical interference and careful often repeated testing has to be done with careful analysis to have confidence in the response recorded in each patient. It can, however, be done reliably after practice in all patients under 60 and in almost all over this age [2]. Each laboratory needs to establish its own technique and normal distribution curve using the equipment available to them just as in any other complex audiological test, for example, ABR so that abnormalities can be documented consistently and reliably. A normal distribution curve is essential for each laboratory when measuring amplitude as well as early and late latencies so that pathological abnormalities on the test are defined. As with all laboratory measurements in the neurotology field, results greater than 2 standard deviations from normal indicate pathology although there is a 1 in 20 chance that such a result is just an extreme or normal [1, 3].

The advantage of sound Ovemps as a stimulus compared to vibration Ovemps is that the side from which any abnormalities arises with sound Ovemps come from the stimulated side, whereas if there is an abnormality with vibration Ovemps, this can be due to abnormalities on either side although more commonly it is the contralateral side which is regarded as abnormal [4].

3. The stapedius reflex. What is it for?

In the human, the footplate of the stapes is directly above and about 3–4 mm lateral to the macula of the saccule [5]. It is visible as a white patch on removal of the stapes footplate. The utricle is close by and slightly above the saccule. Any external sound moving the footplate of the stapes causes a vibratory stimulation of the inner ear fluids. This stimulus reaches the saccule and vibrates the macula before it passes on to the cochlea to be heard.

Until 1964, it was assumed that the stapedius reflex muscle response was present to protect the individual from excessively loud external sounds. At that time, Blair Simmons [6] measured stapedius muscle reflex activity and demonstrated that it was occurring in response to speaking and swallowing. He showed that it began just before the event and ceased just after the event. Extrapolating this finding, it is probable that responses also occur due to biting and chewing food as well as swallowing and belching, blowing the nose, and sniffing, all of which potentially alter the pressure of the middle ear resulting in altered sound transfer to the inner ear and an effect on the cochlea. There is a stapedius reflex response to loud sound but necessarily there is a delay as the sound has to be heard through the cochlea and central processing is necessary for the facial nerve stapedius response. Prior to CT and MRI assessment of the internal auditory canal, the response of stapedius reflex decay in response to sound was one of the tests used to suggest the possible presence of an acoustic neuroma.

The stapedius reflex alters the way the stapes moves [7, 8]. This means that the stimulus received by the inner ear hearing and balance organs differs between when the sound occurs from an internal bodily induced sound stimulus and an external noise when there is no immediate activity of the stapedius muscle. There is a different pattern of vibration of the endolymph beneath the stapes footplate with internally and externally generated sound.

The stapedius reflex response is active immediately and precisely at the commencement of talking and swallowing. The stimulus to the maculae of the saccule and utricle is different when there is an external sound stimulus, and there is no immediate stapedius muscle activity compared to when it is activated due to internal stimulation. This difference allows central differentiation of whether there is an external sound or not. It is essential that both internal and external sound vibration of the perilymph avoids stimulation of the maculae of utricle and saccule resulting in dysfunction of balance activity. Should this occur it would result in instability of the individual potentially making it vulnerable to predation as its instability would reduce effective emergency safety measures such as running, hiding or fighting.

Simmons also speculated that further feedback systems to the inner ear related to hearing and balance would be discovered. The description of the olivocochlear bundle [9, 10] and vestibular efferent systems [11] fulfills his prediction.

A recent, detailed review of effects of loud sounds on the vestibular system was published [12]. It is clear from this, that in animal studies significant damage occurs. Not surprisingly pathological human information is limited. Despite this, it is definite that there is damage to the vestibular system from excessively loud sound, which is due to damage to the maculae of the saccule and utricle particularly the saccule.

A delay occurs between when sound arrives at the inner ear before it is processed in the cochlea, transferred centrally to the brainstem to result in altered stapedius muscle activity *via* the facial nerve. It offers some cochlea protection from unexpected loud sound. There is damage to the otoconia of the maculae not only impairing balance but also resulting in impaired control of reflex responses to sound. The cochlea is less protected than it would otherwise be by the baffle effect of the saccule and macula by otoconia being vibrated and possibly damaged with less afferent reflex responses induced by this stimulation. This will be discussed later. It is suggested that perhaps it is damage to the maculae of the saccule in particular but possibly also the utricle that results in subsequent damage to the cochlea in the 4 K range, which is the site of most noise induced hearing loss.

If an external sound is loud, a stapedius muscle reflex response is generated, necessarily after a short time delay due to processing to determine if it is loud enough to generate the reflex and cochlea brainstem circuitry stimulates the reflex *via* the facial nerve. The stapedius reflex changes the vibratory pattern received by the maculae but as stated there is necessarily a delay between the stimulus and response. If there is a time delay and change in quality of the signal, this indicates that the sound is external rather than a stapedius muscle reflex response to internal sound, which is predicted by and coordinated by the cerebral cortices with the motor activities of swallowing, coughing, etc.

The ability to precisely time the stapedius muscle response resulting in an altered pattern of stimulus to the maculae and cochlea between an internal and external source allows the individual to ascertain if an external sound should be given specific attention and response, while the internal sounds can be recognized and ignored.

4. Threat

Vegetarian animals spend much of their awake hours biting eating and chewing (roughly 80% of the time) and need to be aware of potential predators while continuing to safely and effectively maintain their calorie intake. Because of internal suppression circuitry, the cochlea is able to differentiate these internal noises from potentially dangerous external sounds, while the herbivore is actively biting, chewing or vocalizing. A purpose of this chapter is to explain how this is done.

5. Otoconia. How do they work? What do they do?

The temporal bone consists of calcified collagenous tissue. When undertaking histological study of the inner ear neural structures, it is necessary that the calcium of the temporal bone is dissolved prior to microscopic histology otherwise the calcium blunts the knife preventing satisfactory structural analysis. Unfortunately, the essential histological decalcification preparation means that the calcium in the otoconial system of the maculae is dissolved so it cannot be examined directly at the same time as the vestibular hair cell membranes beneath them. This makes examination to look for structural signs of disease more conjectural. The macula of mammalian saccule and utricle has two types of calcium carbonate otoconia. There are small ones of 2–3 um in diameter and larger ones from 20 to 30 μm in diameter [11]. Due to their inertia, these are vibrated during any head movement including lifting and lowering the head when gravity also affects their motion. When external sound occurs, it also results in movement of the maculae due to the pressure waves caused by the movement of the stapes footplate due to the external sound. They are also moved during the production of internal bodily activity.

DOI: http://dx.doi.org/10.5772/intechopen.111502

6. Internal bodily sounds. How loud are they?

The internal bodily sounds related to speaking consist of a fundamental sound from the larynx adjusted by pharyngeal, oral, lingual, and lip activities. Depending on the frequency of the stimulus and individual resonances of the soft tissues and skull, the amount of vibration of the sounds amplitude varies. These sounds are transferred to the temporal bone (inner ear) in two ways. They are transferred by direct tissue vibration (bone conduction) and also by air conduction particularly the lower frequencies that are heard more clearly through the external auditory canal because of their low frequency characteristics [13]. Sound stimulation of the ears is dependent on the frequency of the sound. Due to the long wavelength of low-frequency sounds, their amplitude is not reduced at corners and little energy is lost. With higher frequencies there is significant attenuation of the sound due to the head shadow effect and therefore, it is heard better in the ear closest to the stimulus [14].

The quality of internal sound changes over time as an animal grows, and it is higher pitched when the animal is younger and smaller and has a lower frequency as the individual grows so that the animal is constantly adjusting responses to maximize the effectiveness of the stimulus detection response of the stapedius reflex in order to suppress dysfunction of the balance system while maximizing detection of external sounds through the ear canal (**Figure 1**).

Surprisingly when measured, internal bodily sounds such as chewing and biting are excessively loud above a level where noise hearing loss would be induced if they were external sounds [13].

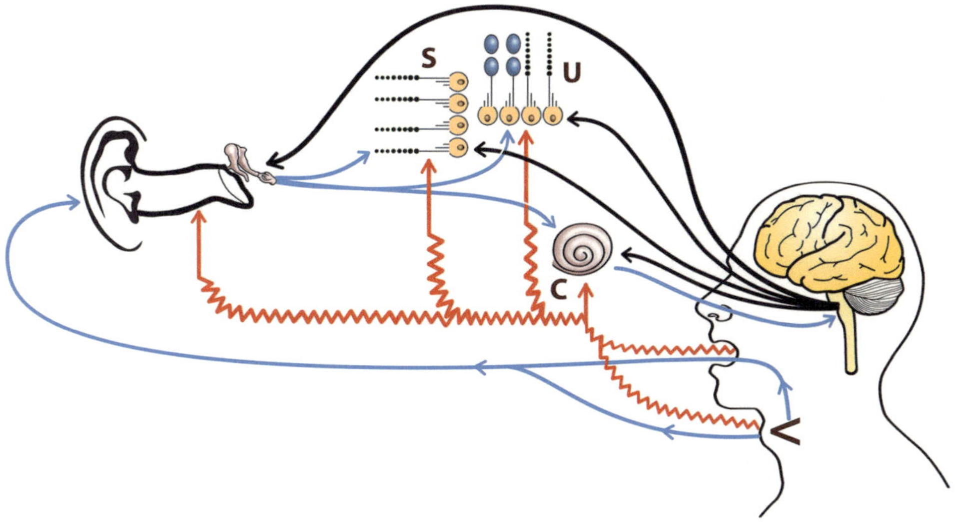

Figure 1.
The black arrows represent efferent pathways from the cerebrum to the stapedius muscle, macular of the utricle, U, macular of the saccular, S, and the cochlear, C. the jagged red lines represent bone—Conducted sound from the larynx during vocalization, and from the mouth during biting, and chewing to the cochlea, utricle, saccule and external auditory canal (EAC). The blue line represents vocalization from the larynx, pharynx and oral cavity via the EAC, through the ossicles to the saccule and utricle. The macula of the saccular, S, diagrammatically shows a cross section of the striola at the line of polarity reversal. The macular of the utricle, U, shows the line of polarity reversal at the junction of the large lateral otoliths with the micro-otoliths of the striola region [15, 16]. The macula of the saccule, S, shows the line of polarity reversal below the microliths of the central striola in the chinchilla (Lysakowski a, personal communication). Taken from Acta Otolaryngologica [13].

Shouting when done as loudly as possible is also excessively loud [13]. In these circumstances why is it that opera singers who are called upon to sing very loudly and practice frequently do not have noise-induced hearing loss. Choir members who are in close proximity to other singers and close to the orchestra do incur noise-induced hearing loss [17]. The explanation for this finding is that the loud internally generated sound in this case from singing is suppressed by internal mechanisms to protect the cochlea.

An extreme example of loud sounds in nature is the male white bellbird, which has been recorded singing with a measured loudness of 125 dB(A); however, birds replace their cochlear hair cells seasonally [18].

Shute [19] proposed many years ago that the saccule could have a hearing function. He ascribed this to nerves traveling to the cochlea *via* the inferior vestibular nerve but bifurcating to travel through the nerve of Oort [20] to reach the basal cochlea as well as the saccular macula. When a sound reaches the saccular macula, it passes by the inferior vestibular nerve centrally but also directly to the cochlea *via* an antidromic reflex through the nerve of Oort.

Excessive noise exposure is recognized as causing measurable vestibular damage. Could cochlea damage be due to lack of protection from otoconial vibration suppression. Should this suggestion be correct, then efforts directed at protection of the vestibular system from excessive noise would be expected also to reduce cochlear damage. Rosen [21] showed that sounds of much lower amplitude than those that cause noise-induced hearing loss result in reduced hearing in older adults exposed to the noises of civilization throughout life such as traffic noise. Wear of the macula system may also occur due to noises of civilization and be why there is gradual deterioration of balance with aging as well as hearing.

Calcium-active drugs have been shown to be associated with improved Cvemps in vestibular migraine. The authors who wrote that article [22] ascribed these improved Cvemp responses to stabilization of brainstem activity by the medication, verapamil; however, it appears logical to this author that verapamil as a calcium-active agent could have acted on the macula otoconia stabilizing them resulting in an improved Cvemp response.

After a patient has head trauma with persistent vestibular complaints, vemps are usually abnormal [2], and a trial of verapamil with sequential repetitive vemps and a quality of life questionnaire would be a worthwhile research project to determine if this type of medication has a place in specifically treating what maybe a macula disorder.

Could treatment to repair malfunctioning otoconia such as calcium-active agents be investigated as a means of restoring otolithic function and perhaps preventing further cochlear damage in individuals who are starting to show signs of noise-induced hearing loss.

Assuming that cochlea injury from excess noise is due to failed otoconial vestibulo-cochlea protection then the symptom of tinnitus which is frequently associated with almost any hearing deficit may well also have induction in the otoconial system as could hyperacusis, which is also frequently associated with hearing loss of any cause including aging and after head trauma.

7. Superior semicircular canal dehiscence syndrome

The sound stimulus for Cvemps and Ovemps is focused and concentrated through the external ear canal. The stimulus for vibration Ovemps applied to the head is a substantially stronger energy stimulus commensurate with the bone conduction sound of speech and chewing. When there is a third window, as in a superior semicircular canals dehiscence syndrome (SSCDS) [23] there is loss of energy from the sound induced C and Ovemp ear canal stimulus which dissipates through the dehiscence. This results in a sub threshold, Cvemp response and an excessively large Ovemp response because of the altered fluid dynamics in the inner ear. There is an apparent reduction in threshold response for air conduction pure tones due to diversion of hydrostatic energy through the third window so less energy reaches the cochlea. The bone conduction stimulus during Ovemp testing is a much larger physical stimulus of the whole temporal bone and is not altered significantly with little energy dissipated if any by the third window. This results in a measured intracochlear conductive hearing deficit during standard pure tone audiometric testing. In the absence of any obvious tympanic membrane or middle ear disorder in the past, this was assumed to be due to otosclerosis despite an intact perhaps raised stapedius reflex threshold prior to the recognition of SSCDS. This concerns the author who wonders over the years how many times low-tone conductive hearing deficits due to SSCDS has been assumed to be due to otosclerosis and the patient has had surgery undertaken. There is a small risk of poor results with otosclerosis surgery and to undertake a procedure for this incorrect diagnosis means that a hearing improvement would not occur but all the risks associated with the surgery exist. Of even more concern is the patient who had revision surgery because of a poor initial operative result because it was due to SSCDS but it was assumed to be a failed "otosclerosis" procedure as complications from revision surgery are much more frequent and serious than with the initial procedure [24, 25].

Radiologically SSCDS is recognized not infrequently in children but it is not symptomatic. This has been put down to very thick dura mater overlying the dehiscence [26]. A more logical explanation is that if an individual has SSCDS at birth or as a small child they adjust, they do not become symptomatic because by being exposed to their own excessively vigorous but to them physiological inner ear fluid movements adjusting "tuning" [8] to the excessive hydrostatically different stimulation of sound and vibration is normal. As an adult after trauma, it is not possible to overcome the sudden substantial physiological dysfunction that occurs with the development of this syndrome and it results in people becoming dizzy with loud sounds and during eating.

There are other third windows disorders where dizziness can be induced by loud sound, and it can occur in tertiary otological syphilis and perilymph fistula. The effects of altered inner ear dynamics in these two disorders on the configuration of Cvemps and Ovemps are dependent on the location in the temporal bone of the third window. Henneberts sign with dizziness due to loud sounds in Ménière's disease is associated with saccular proximity and even attachment to the stapes footplate [27].

8. Cochlea and vestibular efferents. What are they for?

The olivocochlear bundle (OCB) is a poorly understood efferent pathway. How it functions and what it does is still being established [9, 10, 28], which serves to protect the cochlea. It originates in the superior olivary complex in the brainstem and projects to both the ipsilateral and contralateral cochlea. The lateral olivocochlear system has uncrossed synapses ending on type 1 spiral ganglion cells projecting to the inner hair cells. The medial olivocochlear system innervates the outer hair cells and the majority of the fibers project to the contralateral cochlea. Once the efferent reflex is activated, the medial system hyperpolarizes the outer hair cells, which decreases the gain of the cochlea amplifier and sensitivity of the inner hair cells and also reduces the responses of the auditory nerve fibers. Pang [29] has shown that there is an ascending masking effect of about 40 dB due to contraction of the stapedius muscle; this affects the low frequencies to prevent high-frequency attenuation.

There is a system analogous to the olivocochlear bundle efferent system in the macula vestibular system, and it is the vestibular efferent system. During vocalization and chewing, there is otoconial movement due to the vibration of the skull from [13] chewing, biting and vocalizing. The vestibular efferent system suppresses the hair cell stimulation to these expected otoconial vibrations so that specific responses to head and body movement due to gravity change and acceleration/deceleration and head movement are reliably detected without adulteration by extraneous internal stimuli. There is pre-activation of this direct brainstem macula activity and cessation after completion of the task as occurs with the stapedius reflex in response to chewing, biting and talking so that people do not become dizzy.

Activities such as chewing and biting are instructed to occur through standard motor pathways to the appropriate brainstem nuclei and like the stapedius reflex are precisely timed and coordinated with inner ear vestibular and cochlea efferent activity. This maximizes inner ear suppression of inappropriate inadvertent responses in the cochlea and vestibular systems. There is an extremely complex structure of both afferent and efferent vestibular axons with the type 1 and type 2 vestibular hair cells in the maculae [11, 30]. The otoconia are stimulated by internal sounds, swallowing, speaking, etc., but also by movement and gravity, external stimuli which is their main function. One of the main purposes of the complex innervation of the maculae is to allow differentiation of these two stimulus systems, internal and external, so that confusion between the two is avoided and the individual is not destabilized by internal sounds while maintaining perfect balance during movement. Internal sounds cause the otoconia of the maculae to vibrate. When stimulation of the maculae by internal vibration occurs, the stimulus is generalized and similar throughout the maculae, whereas when there is body movement, the complex nature of the orientation of the vestibular hair cells [11, 30] means that certain areas are stimulated while others are not. This optimizes recognition that movement and gravity affect the individual and it is not the effect of internal sounds. Vibration, internal or external, results in movement of otoconia stimulating the vestibular hair cells. As the internal sound of speaking swallowing, etc., is commanded by the cerebral cortex, *via* the brainstem, a vestibular efferent stimulus is sent directly to the maculae to cancel the response to these stimuli due to otoconial vibration caused by internal sounds so that they are available for detection of movement without interference by internal sounds. The brainstem position of the nucleus for vestibular efferents varies depending on taxonomic rank but in all mammals studied it is in close proximity to the facial nucleus making timing for their interrelated activity with the vibratory effect of verbalization, etc. more precisely. It also explains why the distal vestibular efferent neurons synapse on the base of the distal cup of the afferent axon where it surrounds the type 1 vestibular hair cell or directly on the distal afferent axon proximal to the cup as by doing so they are located at a site to most precisely nullify the firing of the afferent neuron in response to internal sound stimulation of the hair cells by the vibrated otoconia. Although the peripheral endings differ in structure in type 2 vestibular hair cells, they also terminate on the basal hair cell and distal peripheral axon, which optimizes there role in suppressing hair cell firing due to internal vibration.

Vestibular hair cells are metabolically very active not only while an individual moves but also due to the effect of internal vibrations while at rest. This high energy demand may explain the need for extra-large mitochondria [31] at the apex of the hair cells to maximize their energy supply from oxidative phosphorylation, because the stereocilia are in a state of almost constant motion except during some periods of sleep when rest and refurbishment occur.

The activities of vocalizing biting and chewing are cerebral cortical tasks undertaken as part of normal human activity while undertaking other more complex tasks requiring significantly more concentration and cerebral cortical activity (thought) but even these simple task can be interrupted immediately by a more urgent need such as an external threat, which indicates that even though simple, these motor tasks at all times are under direct cerebral cortical control and do not function at sub-cortical or thalamic reflex control level.

The function of the semicircular canal system of the inner ear is specifically to maintain the eye fixed on a target while the body and head move. The system can be disconnected urgently if a sudden external stimulus sound or a visual stimulus calls for a rapid head turn and in these circumstances the vestibulo-ocular reflex [VOR] is instantly switched off. There is a coordination with the macula system [32] but this chapter is not the place to discuss the details of how [VOR] function works as it is not specifically related to vibration effects of sounds inside the head and their effect on macula function.

9. Summary

Internal sounds cause the otoconia of the maculae to vibrate. When stimulation of the maculae by internal vibration occurs, the stimulus is generalized and similar throughout the maculae, whereas when there is body movement the complex nature of the orientation of the vestibular hair cells means that certain areas are stimulated, while others are not. This optimizes recognition that movement and gravity affect the individual and it is not the effect of internal sounds. Vibration, internal or external, results in stimulation of the vestibular hair cells. As the internal sound of speaking swallowing, etc., is commanded by the cerebral cortex, *via* the brainstem, a vestibular efferent stimulus is sent directly to the maculae to cancel the activation of vestibular afferent hair cells due to otoconial vibration caused by internal sounds so that they are available for detection of head and body movements without interference by internal sounds. This explains why the distal vestibular efferent neuron synapse on the base of the distal cup of the afferent axon where it surrounds the vestibular hair cell or directly on the distal afferent axon proximal to the cup as by doing so they can most effectively nullify the firing of the afferent neuron in response to internal sound stimulation of the hair cells as this activity is precisely timed to the known internal stimulus to which they also respond. This system is closely analogous to the activity of stapedius muscle reflex in being caused as a response to internal stimuli and perhaps it is more than fortuitous that the brainstem origin of the vestibular efferent system is close to the facial nucleus.

10. Conclusion

This chapter emphasizes the close interaction of the cochlea with the acceleration and gravity detecting macula otoconial vestibular systems of the inner ear. It highlights the complexity and interdependence of the systems. There is need for further studies in this complex field to more fully understand its complex nature, which will hopefully lead to greater understanding of how each system works and to more effective therapy for hearing loss, tinnitus, hyperacusis and imbalance.

Acknowledgements

The author wishes to thank Dr. Art Mallinson for his enthusiasm support and scientific input over the years, Ms. Judy Rousselle for secretarial assistance and Ms. Vicky Earle for diagram production.

Conflict of interest

The author has no conflicts of interest.

Author details

Neil S. Longridge
G & L Diamond Health Care Centre, Vancouver, British Columbia, Canada

*Addreyondence to: nslongridge@hotmail.com

References

[1] Mallinson AI, Longridge NS. Performing and analyzing tool induced cervical and ocular vestibular evoked myogenic potentials in traumatic and nontraumatic vestibular pathology. The Journal of Laryngology and Otology. 2018;**132**(10):896-900

[2] Mallinson AI, Longridge NS. Tone -induced cervical and ocular vestibular-evoked myogenic potentials: Comparing abnormalities in traumatic and non-traumatic vestibular disease. The Journal of Laryngology & Otology. 2018;**132**(10):901-905

[3] Jongkees LB, Phillipzoon. Electronystagmographib analysis of peripheral vertigo. Acta Oto-Laryngologica. 1964;**189**:1-111

[4] Curthoys I. The interpretation of clinical tests of peripheral vestibular function. Laryngoscope. 2012;**122**:1322-1352

[5] Manrique-Huarte R, Zulueta-Santos C, Garaycochea O, Alvarez Linera-Alpert M, Manrique M. Correlation between high-resolution, computed tomography, scan findings and histological findings in human vestibular end organs and surgical implications. Audiol Neurotology. 2020;**25**:42-49. DOI: 10.1159/000504594

[6] Simmons FB. Perceptual theories of middle ear muscle function. The Annals of Otology, Rhinology, and Laryngology. 1964;**73**(3):724-739

[7] Ballantine J, Groves J, editors. Ch 2 physiology of hearing. In: Scott-Brown's Diseases of the Ear Nose and Throat. 4th ed. Vol. 1, Basic Science. London: Butterworths. 1979. p. 87

[8] Longridge NS. Vestibular evoked myogenic potential's: What are they for? An opinion; a hypothesis. Acta Oto-Laryngologica. 2020;**140**(4):255-257. DOI: 10.1080/00016489.2019.1704545

[9] Ciuman RR. The efferent system or olivocochlear function bundle - fine regulator, and protector of hearing perception. International Journal of Biomedical Sciences. 2010;**6**(4):276-288

[10] Laurel AM, Jimenez SV, Delano PH. Olivocochlear efferent effects on perception and behavior. Hearing Research. 2022;**419**. DOI: 10.1016/J. hearse.2021:108207

[11] Lindemann HH. Studies on the Morphology of the Sensory Regions of the Vestibular Apparatus. Berlin, Heidelberg, New York: Springer-Verlaine; 1969

[12] Stewart CE, Holt AG, Altschuler RA, Cacace AT, Hall CD, Murnane OD, et al. Effects of noise exposure on the vestibular system. A systematic review. Frontiers in Neurology. 2020;**11**:593919. DOI: 10.3389/fneurol593919

[13] Longridge NS, Lim A, Mallinson AI, Renshaw J. Vestibular suppression of normal bodily sounds. Acta Oto-Laryngologica. 2020;**140**(5):401-405. DOI: 10.1080/00016489.2020.1723807

[14] Ballantine J, Groves J, editors. Scott-Brown's Diseases of the Ear Nose and Throat. 4th ed. Butterworths. London; Vol. 1 Basic Science, Ch 2 physiology of hearing, p 115-116

[15] Li A, Xue J, Peterson EH. Architecture of the mouse utricle: Macula organization and hair bundle heights. Journal of Neurophysiology. 2008;**99**(2):718-773

[16] Schweitzer FE, Savin D, Luu C, Sultemeier DR, Hoffmann LF.

Distribution of high conductance calcium activated, potassium channels in rat vestibular epithelium. The Journal of Comparative Neurology. 2009;**517**:134-145

[17] Steurer M, Simak S, Denk DM, Kautzsky M. Does choir singing cause noise-induced hearing loss? Audiology. 1998;**37**(1):38-51

[18] Podos J, Cohn-Haft M. 2019 extremely loud mating songs at close range in white bellbirds. Current Biology. 2019;**29**(20):R1068-R1106

[19] Shute C. The anatomy of the eighth cranial nerve in men. Proceeding of the Royal Society of Medicine. 1951;**44**:31-36

[20] Labrousse M, Leveque M, Ouedraogo T, Avisse C, Chays A, Delattre J-F. An anatomical study of the vestibulocochlear anastomosis (anastomosis of Oort) in humans: Preliminary results. Surgical and Radiologic Anatomy. 2005;**27**:238-242. DOI: 10.1007s00276-005-0320-0

[21] Rosen S, Bergman DM, Plester D, El-Monty A, Satti MH. Presbyacusis study of a relatively noise—Free population in the Sudan. The Annals of Otology, Rhinology, and Laryngology. 1962;**71**:727-743. DOI: 1177/000343489466207100313

[22] Liao JJ, Young YH. Vestibular evoked myogenic potential's in basilar artery migraine. The Laryngoscope. 2004;**14**(7):1305-1309

[23] Minor LB. Superior canal dehiscence syndrome. The American Journal of Otology. 2000;**21**(1):9-19

[24] Lundman L, Stromback K, Bjorsne A, Trending J, Redford YD. Otosclerosis revision surgery in Sweden: Hearing outcome, protective factors, and complications. Eur Arch Otorhinolaryngol. 2020;**277**(1):19-29

[25] Picavet V, Govaere F, Fortin G. Superior semicircular canal dehiscence: Prevalence in a population with clinically suspected otosclerosis – Type hearing loss. B-ENT. 2009;**5**:83

[26] Ward BK, Carey JP, Minor LB. Superior canal dehiscence syndrome: Lessons from the first 20 years. Frontiers of Neurology. 2017;**8**:177

[27] Schuknecht HF. Ch 12, Ménière's disease. In: Pathology of the Ear. Vol. 457-465. Cambridge, MOVE THIS. TO LATER. Massachusetts: Harvard University Press; 1974. p. 457

[28] Lapsley ML, Miller JA. How can the auditory efferent system protect our ears from noise induced hearing loss? Let us count the ways. AI Conference Proceedings. 2015;**1703**:090029

[29] Pang XD, Guinean JJ. Effects of stapedius muscle contraction on the masking of auditory nerve responses. The Journal of the Acoustical Society of America. 1997;**102**(6):276-288

[30] Lindemann HH. Regional differences in structure of the vestibular sensory regions. The Journal of Laryngology and Otology. 1969;**83**(1):1-17

[31] Vranceanu F, Perkins GG, Terada M, Chidavaenzi RL, Ellisman MH, Lysakowski A. Striated organelle a cytoskeletal structure positioned to modulate hair-cell transduction. The Proceedings of the National Academy of Sciences. 2012;**109**(12):4473-4478. DOI: 10.1073/Pas.1101003109

[32] Longridge NS, Mallinson AI, Pothier DD. Do otoliths modulate caloric response? What do vemps and CDP measure? What do these tests tell us? The Journal of Otolaryngology-ENT Research. 2015;**3**(2):1-5

Chapter 4

Role of cVEMP in Management of Balance Disorders

Renu Rajguru

Abstract

Balance disorders may occur in a multitude of ENT-related diseases, thus making a correct diagnosis is challenging. In the last few decades, there has been a paradigm shift in the diagnostics of balance disorders due to the availability of better objective modalities that allow the assessment of different components of the complex vestibular labyrinth with relative ease. With the advent of vestibular-evoked myogenic potentials (VEMP) since the last few decades, it is possible to test otolith organs in isolation and objectively. This chapter will discuss the procedure, physiological basis, and effectiveness of cervical VEMP in the evaluation of saccular function in patients suffering from balance disorders.

Keywords: saccular dysfunction, vestibular-evoked myogenic potentials, vestibular neuritis, superior semicircular canal dehiscence syndrome, Meniere's disease, posterior canal benign paroxysmal positional vertigo

1. Introduction

Balance disorders are one of the most common presentations to otolaryngology clinic. Inability to maintain balance or occurrence of vertigo has a considerable impact on social and working life. Imbalance is one of the most common symptoms which patients experience at some time or the other in their lifetime, with a lifetime prevalence of about 30% and an annual incidence that increases with age [1]. Despite this high prevalence and burden of disease, diagnosing the cause of imbalance remains a considerable challenge as the pathology may involve many sensory organs.

Most patients with balance disorders are uncertain who to consult, because their problem lies in between the specialties of neurology, otolaryngology, and in some cases, ophthalmology, general/internal medicine, endocrinology, or psychiatry. Imbalance, whether episodic or chronic, causes significant deterioration in the quality of life of a person and can cause anxiety, depression, reduced physical activity, and possible inability to work. In elderly population, falls due to imbalance add to existing morbidity to a great extent [2].

In the last few decades, availability of better objective modalities which help in assessing different components of complex vestibular labyrinth with relative ease have led to better diagnostics of balance disorders, and now precise localization of the vestibular disorders possible. These tests are rapid, reliable, and effective in diagnosing balance disorders.

The vestibular system consists of the three semicircular canals (lateral, superior, and posterior) and otolith organs (saccule and utricle). The majority of the clinical vestibular function tests for imbalance such as the caloric test, head impulse test, Dix-Hallpike test, supine roll test, subjective visual vertical, VNG, rotational tests mainly test the semicircular canals. But with the advent of vestibular-evoked myogenic potentials (VEMP), it is possible to test otolith organs separately and objectively. Various studies showed that high intensity sound stimulus resulted in activation of vestibule apart from stimulating cochlea and generated electromyographic reflexes in many muscles including sternocleidomastoid (SCM) and extraocular muscles. It was also possible to easily record these electromyographic reflexes with surface electrodes placed on SCM. The electromyographic reflexes recorded over SCM are called cervical VEMP or cVEMP, and they record sacculo-collic reflex, and those on the extra ocular muscles are called ocular VEMP or oVEMP and they record utriculo-collic reflex [3]. This chapter shall dwell upon cVEMP primarily.

2. Physiological basis of VEMP

The physiology of cVEMP generation has been hypothesized based on tendency of the animals to look in the direction of sound. Evolution has proved that vestibular system evolved earlier than the cochlear system. In reptiles and marine animals, the vestibular system served the purpose of hearing too. The saccule, which is part of otolithic organ, has remnants of these hearing receptors. These are transmitted *via* the inferior vestibular nerve, which eventually results in reflex turning of head in the direction of sound. This reflex is being commonly employed in our day-to-day clinical practice too. Turning of head in the direction of sound is a complex movement, which involves integration of auditory stimulus with vestibulo-spinal pathway. This is achieved by reflex inhibition of contraction of ipsilateral SCM muscle and contraction of contralateral SCM muscle, which results in turning of head toward the direction of sound. Cervical VEMP records the inhibitory signals of sacculo-collic reflex being generated from ipsilateral SCM in response to stimulation of saccule due to sound as it is situated very close to the oval window which itself is stimulated by sound. The reflex pathway is through inferior vestibular nerve (IVN) and the central nervous system (CNS), and is picked up by electrodes placed on ipsilateral SCM [4]. The neural pathway of cVEMP generation following presentation of sound stimulus given through insert earphones on the side to be tested is explained in the subsequent paragraph:

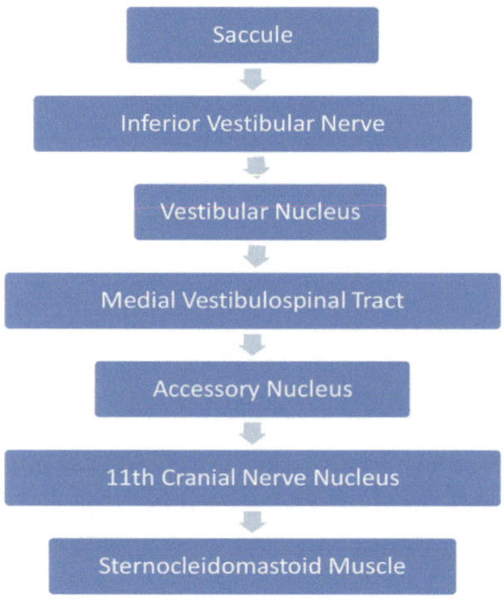

This recording is then used in the evaluation of saccular function in diagnosis of balance disorders by analyzing cVEMP parameters (threshold, latency of P13 and N23 peak, and the amplitude). The other parameters that can be derived from these basic parameters are: the interaural amplitude difference ratio that is calculated by dividing the interaural difference of P13-N23 interamplitude by the sum of P13-N23 interamplitude of both ears, P13-N23 interlatency, P13-N23 interamplitude, and absolute interear difference [5].

3. Methodology

The test is usually done either in the sitting position or in the lying down position. When done in sitting position, the patient is made to turn his head to contralateral side from the ear being tested. The contraction of SCM muscle can also be monitored objectively by keeping inflated cuff of sphygmomanometer between shoulder and mandible and the patient is asked to maintain pressure at a constant level, maintaining a tonicity of SCM at 30–75 *M*v [5]. While conducting the test in the lying down position, the patient may be made to lie down with head raised to about 30 degree without support and chin not touching the chest, and head turned contralaterally to the ear being tested to activate maximally the SCM muscle ipsilateral to the stimulation. However, it can be done in recumbent and prone positions too with head lifted or head turned [5].

There are no specific devices to be used in VEMP testing, and most of the centers use the Brainstem Evoked Response Audiometry (BERA) or Auditory Brainstem Response (ABR) equipment with special VEMP software to record these responses.

The electrode placed on the middle one-third of ipsilateral sternocleidomastoid muscle to be tested is called positive or active electrode, that on the sternal head of sternocleidomastoid muscle is called reference or inactive electrode and the one on forehead is called ground electrode (**Figure 1**). The stimulus in the form of tone bursts at an intensity of 98 dB nHL (120 dBSPL), using a 5 dB up, 10 dB down-step procedure is presented to the test ear by insert ear phone with foam ear tips. The tone bursts are given at 500 Hz as 200 stimuli of 0.2 milli-sec each [5]. The potentials are then recorded with standard disposable, self-adhesive surface electrodes. The electrode impedance is kept within optimum level by using conduction gel in all cases.

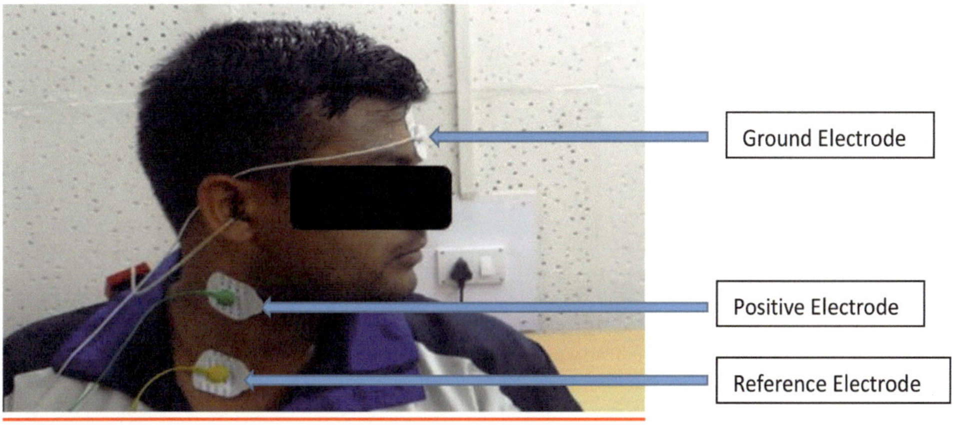

Figure 1.
Placement of electrodes.

The results are obtained from the software in the form of a graph showing latency on the X-axis measured in milli-seconds and amplitude on the Y-axis measured as microvolts. The first positive peak, that is, downward deflection is termed as P13 wave and is recorded at 13 millisec. N23 wave is the first negative peak and is recorded at 23 milli-sec. Both waves are recorded for each ear separately (**Figures 2** and **3**) [4]. The summation potentials recorded are then analyzed. The presence of cVEMP is confirmed by doing three consecutive summation potential recordings. Any prolongation of the positive peak or increase in latency or decrease in amplitude means that

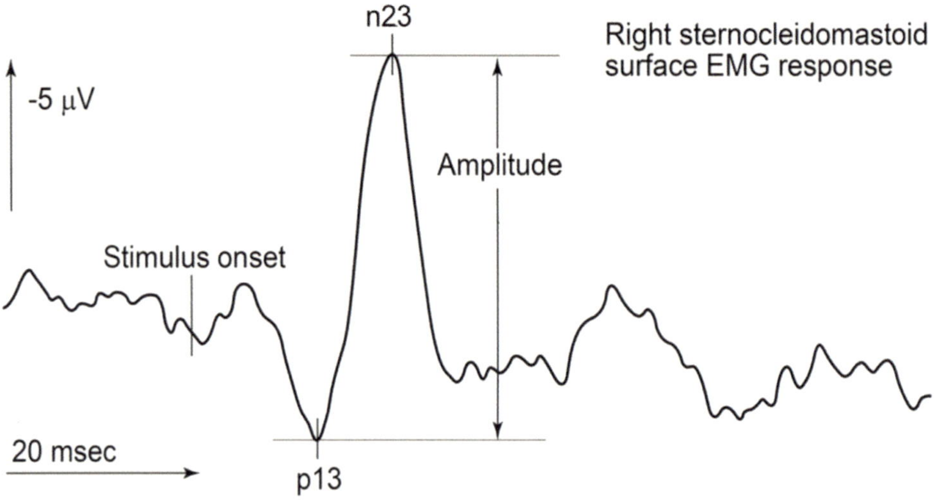

Figure 2.
cVEMP waveform showing latency and amplitude, P13 being the first positive peak and N23 the first negative peak.

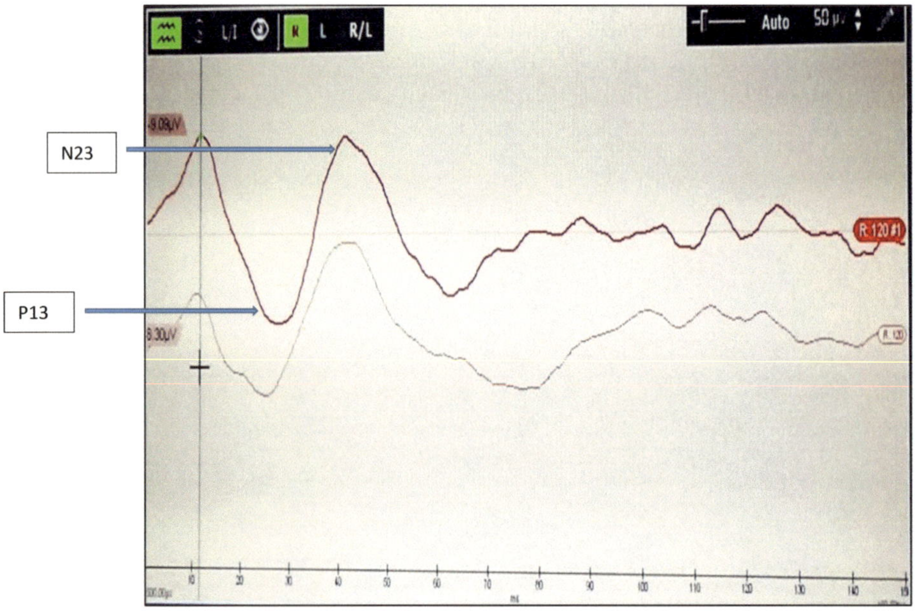

Figure 3.
cVEMP waveform as seen on the computer screen showing P13 and N 23 waves.

cVEMP is abnormal, and that there is saccular dysfunction. The interaural difference of latency from the peaks is associated with the speed of neuronal conduction, and any alteration in this speed may be a result of neurological disease process. The basic cVEMP parameters are threshold, latency of P13 and N23 peak and their amplitude. Other parameters that can be derived from these basic parameters are the interaural amplitude difference ratio which is calculated by dividing the interaural difference of P13-N23 interamplitude by the sum of P13-N23 interamplitude of both ears.

4. Clinical applications

4.1 Benign paroxysmal positional vertigo

BPPV occurs due to the displacement of calcium-carbonate crystals or otoconia within the fluid-filled semicircular canals of the inner ear. These otoconia are essential for the proper functioning of the utricle of the otolithic membrane by helping deflect the hair cells within the endolymph, which relays positional changes of the head, including tilting, turning, and linear acceleration [6]. As cVEMP primarily detects saccular dysfunction, hence it is possible that the cVEMP parameters may be normal in BPPV. But there are studies which have shown abnormal cVEMP parameters in cases of BPPV. Yang et al. in their study found an increase in VEMP latencies, a finding which was also demonstrated by Godha et al. in their study. Godha et al. also showed high specificity and low sensitivity of VEMP for diagnosing BPPV [7, 8].

4.2 Vestibular neuritis

The usual symptoms of vestibular neuritis (VN) are imbalance, vertigo, nausea, and vomiting, and these symptoms are present in many other clinical conditions such as labyrinthitis, Menier's disease etc. To establish that these symptoms are due to inflammation of the vestibular nerve, complete or partial unilateral loss of vestibular function needs to be established. This cannot be done by Caloric test or head impulse test as they assess only lateral semicircular canal function and hence, these tests would be normal in patients of VN, thus creating a diagnostic dilemma. Hence, VEMP especially oVEMP which tests superior vestibular nerve function is useful for the diagnosis of VN patients. But in some cases, cVEMP parameters are also found to be abnormal. In a study by Tripathi et al., out of the 10 VN patients, cVEMP was bilaterally normal in seven patients indicating that they had superior vestibular neuritis, but in three patients, they found reduced amplitude in the effected ears indicating inferior vestibular neuritis (IVN) in these patients [9]. Halmagayi et al. published a similar study for the diagnosis of IVN [10]. Murofushi et al. in their study found normal latencies in VN patients and prolonged latencies only in retrolabyrinthine lesions [11]. Nola et al. in their study found that superior VN patients showed normal amplitude and latency on both sides, but IVN patients showed abnormal parameters which changed to normal once the acute attack was over [12]. This study suggested use of VEMP as a screening test for VN. Monstad et al. also reported similar findings in their case series [13].

4.3 Ménière's disease (MD)

The most supported pathophysiological mechanism in MD is endolymphatic hydrops, characterized by excessive endolymphatic accumulation in the cochlea and vestibule [14]. The most commonly affected inner ear structures in MD are cochlea and the saccule, followed by utricle and semicircular canals [15, 16]. Hence, cVEMP parameters, if abnormal, support the diagnosis of MD in case of diagnostic dilemma. Saccular dysfunction causing saccular hydrops can cause cVEMP parameters to be abnormal in the effected ear, which may either be absent or may show reduced amplitude. Reduced peak-to-peak amplitudes as compared with controls were also found by Zuniga et al. and Salviz et al. in their respective studies [17, 18].

Absent or reduced cVEMP responses were also found by Angeli and Goncalves in 74% of the patients with active MD and 50% patients with stable MD [19].

Thus, cVEMP can be used to identify patients whose symptoms are suggestive, but not diagnostic for MD, and also to track saccular function over time. In case of unilateral MD, cVEMP can also be used to monitor the asymptomatic ear to know whether that ear will develop MD or nor not [20]. A study published by Rauch et al. in 2004 found VEMP parameters to be altered in about 94% of the patients with MD in the affected side in terms of increase in frequency thresholds between 250 and 2000 Hz. Also, about 27% of the asymptomatic ears with unilateral MD had altered cVEMP parameters. Thus, VEMP was found to be not only a diagnostic method for endolymphatic hydrops in initial stages, but also a prognostic factor for bilateral involvement in MD [21].

4.4 Superior semicircular canal dehiscence syndrome (SCD)

SCD is caused due to dehiscence of bone over superior semicircular canal, which creates a third mobile window in the labyrinth. Loud sounds or pressure changes in external auditory canal or middle ear may cause imbalance, vertigo, hearing loss, autophony, or pulsatile tinnitus as this third window serves as a low-resistance pathway for transmission of low-frequency sound energy through the labyrinth. This also lowers the threshold required for generation of cVEMP to a large extent and raises

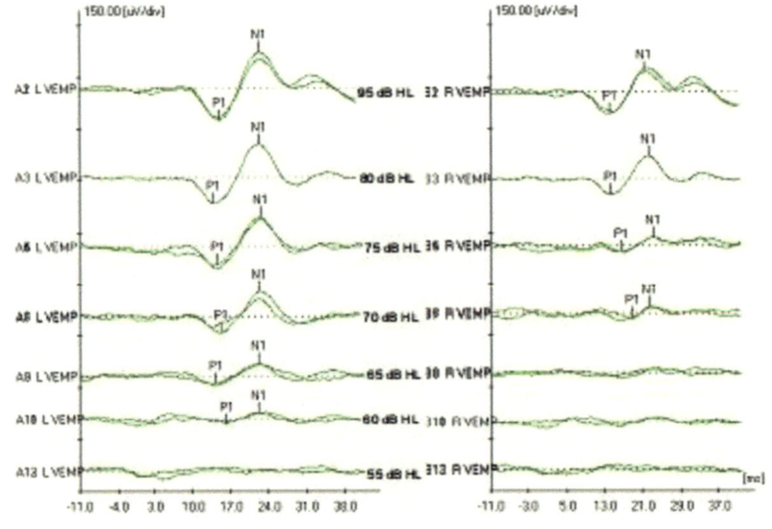

Figure 4.
cVEMP with recordable P13 and N23 waves obtained in a patient with left SCD at 60 dB.

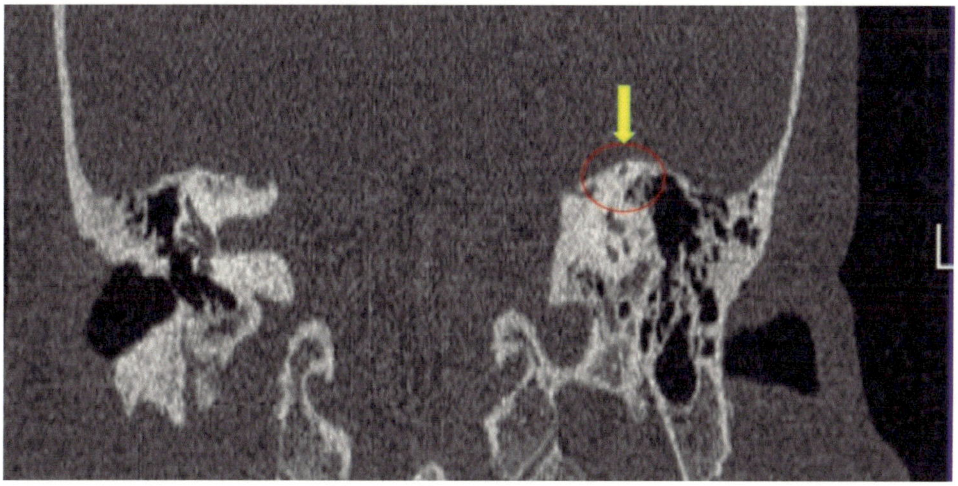

Figure 5.
HRCT temporal bone of the same patient confirming the diagnosis of left SCD.

the resultant amplitude (**Figure 4**). Though the confirmatory investigation for SCD is HRCT temporal bone, it may over estimate the size of the dehiscence or can falsely detect dehiscence in patients with very thin bony covering, resulting in erroneous diagnosis of SCD. VEMP is uniquely suited for identification of SCD as it can be used to detect whether it is the dehiscence which is causing pathological pressure transmission in the vestibular labyrinth.

SCD patients show reduced threshold and high amplitude in the effected ears, and normal parameters in contralateral healthy ears. Tripathi et al. in their study found the threshold to be as low as 50 dB [9]. The diagnosis of these cases was confirmed by doing HRCT temporal bone and they found dehiscence of superior semicircular canal in the images obtained (**Figure 5**). Similar findings were seen in studies done by Streubel et al. [22]. Also, Zhou et al. in their study of 65 patients, obtained abnormally low VEMP thresholds and found VEMP to be highly sensitive and specific for SCD, possibly better than CT [23]. Welgampola et al. in their study of 12 SCD cases found VEMP thresholds to be pathologically lowered in all, which normalized after corrective surgery [24].

4.5 Vestibular schwannoma

Vestibular schwannoma (VS), formerly known as acoustic neuroma, is a benign slow growing tumor that develops from Schwann cells of the vestibular nerve. The tumor arises within the internal auditory canal and grows into the cerebello-pontine angle, resulting in unilateral/asymmetric hearing loss and/or tinnitus and loss of balance. It is third most common intracranial benign tumor after meningioma and pituitary adenoma [25]. As the symptoms are subtle and varied, early detection of the tumor is sometimes difficult. Though the investigation of choice for the diagnosis of VS is MRI, it is costly and every suspected patient may not afford it, so other diagnostic modalities also play an important role in diagnosing vestibular schwannomas.

Knowing that VEMP neural pathways involve the inferior portion of the vestibular nerve, this diagnostic method can also be used to help in the diagnosis of VS. Murofushi et al. in their study published in 1998 noticed changes in VEMP parameters in 80% of their vestibular schwannoma patients [26]. Takeichi et al. published a study in 2001 in which they found alteration in VEMP parameters in 72% of their vestibular schwannoma patients [27].

Chiarovano et al. in their study published in 2014 to evaluate the role of Cervical and Ocular Vestibular-Evoked Myogenic Potentials in the assessment of patients with vestibular schwannomas conducted all oto-neurologic tests on 37 of the 63 unoperated patients of VS and made some important observations after analyzing their data which modified their clinical practice [28]. They found that inferior vestibular nerve (abnormal cVEMPs: 62%) was less frequently involved in the disease process as compared to the superior vestibular nerve (abnormal oVEMPs: 76%). Also, 16% percent of these patients had abnormal VEMP but normal hearing and normal caloric test. Thus, it is possible to use VEMP as a diagnostic test (as it may be the only abnormal vestibular finding) and also as a modality for follow up.

From then onwards they started doing VEMPs systematically in patients suffering from vertigo or imbalance and an MRI centered on the IAC was requested in the case of isolated abnormal cervical or ocular VEMPs. They also found that cVEMPs and oVEMPs allowed the evaluation of the effects of treatment on VS patients who had undergone stereotactic radiosurgery. They concluded that the role of the VEMPs in VS is not only in the diagnosis, but is also in assessment of the function of the superior and inferior vestibular nerves prior to surgery and/or microradiosurgery. VEMP testing as a baseline test for patients undergoing surgery and/or microradiosurgery had two distinct advantages: First, it served as a guide to how to assess residual vestibular function so that vestibular rehabilitation could be planned post-treatment, and, second, it helped to determine if the cause of imbalance was vestibular decompensation or further compromise of vestibular function and accordingly rehabilitation was planned. Though VEMPs can contribute to the diagnosis of vestibular tumors and serve as an excellent screening tool, they cannot be used as the sole diagnostic method, because they only assess the function of the inferior vestibular nerve. But when performed together with MRI, the ABR, audiometry and caloric test, they help in the exact location of the tumor in the vestibular pathways.

4.6 Perilymphatic fistula

A perilymphatic fistula is an abnormal communication between the perilymph-filled inner ear to outside, which causes perilymph to leak from the cochlea or vestibule, most commonly through the round or oval window, resulting in cochlear and vestibular symptoms [29]. The audiovestibular symptoms of perilymph fistula mimic various other conditions, which lack precise diagnostic tools such as Meniere's disease, superior or posterior canal dehiscence, endolymphatic hydrops, Eustachian tube dysfunction, vestibular migraine, mal de debarquement, and persistent postural-perceptual dizziness. For decades, the gold standard for diagnosis of a perilymph fistula has been exploratory tympanotomy with intra-operative visualization of perilymph leakage with subsequent improvement in symptoms after the leak has been repaired. However, this test is not only invasive but also subjective as no established criteria exist for what constitutes a perilymphatic leak on observation. In 2006, Modugno et al. published a study in which VEMP testing was used for the diagnosis of endolymphatic fistula cases [30]. They reported four cases in which VEMP response thresholds were reduced with stimuli in the frequency of 500 Hz.

The VEMP thresholds are lowered due to third window effect which reduces the impedance, similar to superior semicircular canal dehiscence. So cVEMP can be used as a screening tool prior to other sophisticated imaging modalities such as CT and MRI with axial and coronal Constructive Interference in Steady State (CISS), also called Fast Imaging Employing Steady-State Acquisition (FIESTA) or Magnetic Resonance Perfusion (MRP) sequence [29].

4.7 Monitoring after treatment with intratympanic gentamicin

In Ménière's disease, those cases with intolerable vertigo and resistance to clinical treatment, administration of intratympanic gentamicin is done in an attempt to reduce vertigo symptoms in these patients [31]. After this therapy, VEMP can be used to confirm if the gentamicin dose employed was enough to cause damage to the vestibular cells. In 2002, De Waele et al. showed that 92% of the patients submitted to intratympanic injection of gentamicin had absent responses in VEMP testing [32].

5. Clinical applications in pediatric population

Balance disorders in children due to vestibular disorders are not well documented as compared to the adult population. It is so because clinicians often rely on parent's inputs to screen for vestibular dysfunction, especially when the child is too young to verbalize their symptoms. Vestibular function testing in children is not an easy task as they may not self-report or even be aware that their symptoms are abnormal. Also, their short attention span makes any test more challenging. The prevalence of balance and vestibular disorders in children is estimated between 0.45 and 5.3%, with a slightly higher prevalence in females over males, which tends to rise with age [33, 34]. VEMP forms an important part of pediatric vestibular testing battery right from the birth of the child. Early development of the Vestibular Colic Reflex facilitates the ability to use cVEMP testing in children younger than 12 months. Pediatric normative amplitude ranges are approximately 208.5 to 285.00 μV, and normative cVEMP threshold responses are at approximately 105 to 110 dB SPL [35, 36].

As in the adults, cVEMPs are considered abnormal if responses are absent or low in amplitude; however, with third window disorders, such as enlarged vestibular aqueduct or superior canal dehiscence, large amplitudes and low thresholds are considered abnormal.

VEMP testing in children provides the clinician with diagnostic information about otolith function that cannot be identified by other tests. It is well received by children because the testing procedure does not require that they be in the dark, does not induce symptoms of dizziness, and they can sit with or close to their parent. Also it is quick, painless and non-invasive.

5.1 Neonatal vestibular screening

Verrecchia et al. in their pilot study published in 2019 used VEMP for newborn vestibular screening alongside the regional newborn hearing screening program. They used bone-conducted stimuli to test VEMP. The tonicity of neck muscles was maintained by resting the infants unconstrained in their parents′ arms, while the operator supported the infant's head with his hand. Performed this way, they found VEMP protocol to be highly viable and reproducible. They concluded that VEMP can be used for large-scale assessment of vestibular function in infants if integrated into the newborn hearing screening program [37].

5.2 Cochlear implant surgery

Assessment of vestibular function is also done in children pre- and post-cochlear implantation. Otolith damage may occur during cochlear implant surgery as saccule lies very close to the insertion pathway of the implant's electrode array. cVEMP responses are absent in about 40 to 80% of children following cochlear implantation. Wolter et al. in their retrospective study compared 35 children with CI failure to 165 children who did not experience CI failure. Saccular function was assessed by VEMP. They found that a greater proportion of children with CI failure had abnormal saccular function compared to those without CI failure (81 vs. 46%, $p = 0.003$). They suggested early identification and treatment of such impairments so as to avoid or delay implant failures and prevent children from experiencing periods of sound deprivation that could impact speech and language acquisition [38].

In addition VEMP has also been used to demonstrate vestibular dysfunction in conditions such as autism and spastic cerebral palsy [39, 40].

6. Conclusion

VEMP is a relatively newer vestibular function test, which can test otolith organs in isolation and objectively. oVEMP is the objective test for utricle and superior vestibular nerve, whereas cVEMP tests saccule and the inferior vestibular nerve. As it does not induce vertigo, it is more acceptable and comfortable for the patients. It is a non-invasive test and the electromyographic potentials are stable and repeatable, can be documented, and reproduced objectively. The cost is very less as it uses hardware of ABR testing. It is also an excellent tool for screening of vestibular system in newborns and has extensive applications in pediatric population. These advantages make it an excellent tool in management of vestibular disorders. However, in many clinical conditions it cannot be used as the sole diagnostic modality, but is a complementary test, which when done along with other investigative procedures, points to a diagnosis in case of balance disorders.

Author details

Renu Rajguru
Department of ENT, All India Institute of Medical Sciences, Raipur, India

*Address all correspondence to: renurajguru@yahoo.com

References

[1] Strupp M. Challenges in neuro-otology. Frontiers in Neurology. 2010;**1**(121):1-2

[2] Bronstein AM. Evaluation of balance. In: Gleeson M, editor. Scott-Brown's Otorhinolaryngology, Head and Neck Surgery. 7th ed. Hodder Arnold: CRC Press; 2008. pp. 3706-3747

[3] Rauch SD. Vestibular evoked myogenic potentials. Current Opinion in Otolaryngology & Head and Neck Surgery. 2006;**14**(5):299-304

[4] Cal R, Bahmad F Jr. Vestibular evoked myogenic potentials: An overview. Brazilian Journal of Otorhinolaryngology. 2009;**75**(3):456-462

[5] Isaradisaikul S, Navacharoen N, Hanprasertpong C, Kangsanarak J. Cervical vestibular-evoked myogenic potentials: Norms and protocols. International Journal of Otolaryngology. 2012;**2012**:913515. DOI: 10.1155/2012/913515 Epub 2012 Apr 8

[6] Epley JM. New dimensions of benign paroxysmal positional vertigo. Otolaryngology and Head and Neck Surgery 1979. 1980;**88**(5):599-605

[7] Yang WS, Kim SH, Lee JD, Lee WS. Clinical significance of vestibular evoked myogenic potentials in benign paroxysmal positional vertigo. Otorhinolaryngology. 2008;**29**(8):1162-1166

[8] Godha S, UpadhyayMundra A, Mundra RK, Bhalot L, Singh A. VEMP: An objective test for diagnosing the cases of BPPV. Indian Journal of Otolaryngology and Head and Neck Surgery. 2020;**72**(2):251-256. DOI: 10.1007/s12070-020-01802-3 Epub 2020 Feb 27

[9] Tripathi S, Rajguru R, Gupta AK, Patil B. Is cervical vestibular evoked myogenic potentials an effective tool for the evaluation of saccular function in patients suffering from peripheral vertigo? An analytical study. Indian Journal of Otology. 2020;**26**:247-253

[10] Halmagayi GM, Aw ST, Karlberg M, Curthoys IS, Todd MJ. Inferior vestibular neuritis. Annals of the New York Academy of Sciences. 2002;**956**:306-313

[11] Murofushi T, Shimizu K, Takegoshi H, Cheng PW. Diagnostic value of prolonged latencies in the VEMP. Archives of Otolaryngology - Head and Neck Surgery. 2001;**127**(9):1069-1072

[12] Nola G, Guastini L, Crippa B, Deiana M, Mora R, Ralli G. Vestibular evoked myogenic potential in vestibular neuritis. European Archives of Otorhinolaryngology. 2011;**268**(11):1671-1677

[13] Monstad P, Okstad S, Mygland A. Inferior vestibular neuritis: 3 cases with clinical features of acute vestibular neuritis, normal calorics but indication of saccular failure. BMC Neurology. 2006;**6**:45

[14] Gürkov R, Pyykö I, Zou J, Kentala E. What is Menière's disease? A contemporary re-evaluation of endolymphatic hydrops. Journal of Neurology. 2016;**263**:71-81. Published online 2016 Apr 15. DOI: 10.1007/s00415-015-7930-1

[15] Lopez-Escamez JA, Carey J, Chung W-H, Goebel JA, et al. Diagnostic criteria for Meniere's disease. Journal of Vestibular Research. 2015;**25**:1-7

[16] Okuno T, Sando I. Localisation, frequency, and severity of endolymphatic

hydrops and the pathology of the labyrinthine membrane in Meniere's disease. Annals of Otology, Rhinology & Laryngology. 1987;**96**:438-445

[17] Zuniga MG, Janky KL, Schubert MC, Carey JP. Can vestibular evoked myogenic potentials help differentiate Meniere disease from vestibular migraine? Otolaryngology–Head and Neck Surgery. 2012;**146**(5):788-796

[18] Salviz M, Yuce T, Acar H, Taylan I, Yuceant GA, Karatas A. Diagnostic value of vestibular evoked myogenic potentials in Meniere disease and vestibular migraine. Journal of Vestibular Research. 2016;**25**(5-6):261-266

[19] Angeli SI, Goncalves S. Cervical VEMP tuning changes by Meniere's disease stages. Laryngoscope Investigative Otolaryngology. 2019;**4**(5):543-549

[20] Van Tilburg MJ, Herrmann BS, Guinan JJ Jr, Rauch SD. Serial cVEMP testing is sensitive to disease progression in Meniere patients. Otology & Neurotology. 2016;**37**(10):1614-1619

[21] Rauch SD, Zhou G, Kujawa SG, Guinan JJ, Herrmann BS. Vestibular evoked myogenic potentials show altered tuning in patients with Meniere's disease. Otology & Neurotology. 2004;**25**(3):333-338

[22] Streubel SO, Cremer PD, Carey JP, Weg N, Minor LB. Vestibular evoked myogenic potentials in the diagnosis of superior semicircular canal dehiscence syndrome. Acta Oto-Laryngologica. Supplementum. 2001;**545**:41-49

[23] Zhou G, Gopen Q, Poe DS. Clinical and diagnostic characterisation of canal dehiscence syndrome: A great otologic mimicker. Otology & Neurotology. 2007;**28**:920-926

[24] Welgampola MS, Myrie OA, Minor LB, Carey JP. VEMP thresholds normalize on plugging superior semicircular canal dehiscence. Neurology. 2008;**70**(6):464-4720

[25] Ostrom QT, Gittleman H, Liao P, et al. CBTRUS statistical report: Primary brain and other central nervous system tumors diagnosed in the United States in 2010-2014. Neuro-Oncology. 2017;**19**(suppl_5):v1-v88

[26] Murofushi T, Matsuzaki M, Mizuno M. Vestibular evoked myogenicpotentials in patients with acoustic neuromas. Archives of Otolaryngology–Head & Neck Surgery. 1998;**124**(5):509-512

[27] Takeichi N, Sakamoto T, Fukuda S, et al. Vestibular evoked myogenicpotentials (VEMP) in patients with acoustic neuromas. Auris, Nasus, Larynx. 2001;**28**(Suppl):S39-S41

[28] Chiarovano E, Darlington C, Vidal P-P, Lamas G, de Waele C. The role of cervical and ocular vestibular evoked myogenic potentials in the assessment of patients with vestibular schwannomas. PLoS One. 2014;**9**(8):e105026. DOI: 10.1371/journal.pone.0105026

[29] Sarna B, Abouzari M, Merna C, Jamshidi S, Saber T, Djalilian HR. Perilymphatic fistula: A review of classification, etiology, diagnosis, and treatment. Frontiers in Neurology. 2020;**11**:1046. DOI: 10.3389/fneur.2020.01046

[30] Modugno GC, Magnani G, Brandolini C, Savastio G, Pirodda A. Could vestibular evoked myogenic potentials (VEMPs) also be useful in the diagnosis of perilymphatic fistula? European Archives of Oto-Rhino-Laryngology. 2006;**263**(6):552-555. DOI: 10.1007/s00405-006-0008-z Epub 2006 Feb 16

[31] Carey JP. Intratympanic gentamicin for the treatment of Meniere's disease and other forms of peripheral vertigo. Otolaryngologic Clinics of North America. 2004;**37**(5):1075-1090

[32] DeWaele C, Menguenni R, Freyess G, et al. Intratympanic gentamicin injections for Meniere's disease: Vestibular hair cell impairment and regeneration. Neurology. 2002;**59**(9):1442-1444

[33] O'Reilly RC, Morlet T, Nicholas BD, et al. Prevalence of vestibular and balance disorders in children. Otology & Neurotology. 2010;**31**(09):1441-1444

[34] Li CM, Hoffman HJ, Ward BK, Cohen HS, Rine RM. Epidemiology of dizziness and balance problems in children in the United States: A population-based study. The Journal of Pediatrics. 2016;**17**:1240-1270

[35] Janky KL, Rodriguez AI. Quantitative vestibular function testing in the Pediatric population. Seminars in Hearing. 2018;**39**(3):257-274. DOI: 10.1055/s-0038-1666817 Epub 2018 Jul 20

[36] Maes L, De Kegel A, Van Waelvelde H, Dhooge I. Rotatory and collic vestibular evoked myogenic potential testing in normal-hearing and hearing-impaired children. Ear and Hearing. 2014;**35**(02):e21-e32

[37] Verrecchia L, Karpeta N, Westin M, Johansson A, Aldenklint S, Brantberg K, et al. Methodological aspects of testing vestibular evoked myogenic potentials in infants at universal hearing screening program. Scientific Reports. 2019;**9**(1):17225. DOI: 10.1038/s41598-019-53143-z

[38] Wolter NE, Gordon KA, Papsin BC, Cushing SL. Vestibular and balance impairment contributes to cochlear implant failure in children. Otology & Neurotology. 2015;**36**(6):1029-1034

[39] Oster LM, Zhou G. Balance and vestibular deficits in pediatric patients with autism spectrum disorder: An underappreciated clinical aspect. Autism Research and Treatment. 2022;**2022**:7568572. DOI: 10.1155/2022/7568572

[40] Akbarfahimi N, Hosseini SA, Rassafiani M, et al. Assessment of the saccular function in children with spastic cerebral palsy. Neurophysiology. 2016;**48**:141-149. DOI: 10.1007/s11062-016-9580-z

Chapter 5

Otoneurological Evaluation and Rehabilitative Considerations after Head Trauma

Maria Cristina Alves Corazza, Luíza Alves Corazza and Júlia Alves Corazza

Abstract

Head injuries due to traffic accidents, falls, gunshots and blows in sports fights, among others, with or without a skull or petrosal fractures, can lead to a Traumatic Labyrinth Concussion (TLC), defined as a disorder of the peripheral vestibular system comprising vestibular, auditory and neurovegetative signs and symptoms, which can persist for weeks or months after a traumatic injury. It is often accompanied by central nervous system (CNS) concussion, manifested by objective symptoms such as tachycardia, headache, thermoregulatory instability and mydriasis; and subjective complaints such as emotional disorders, memory loss, visual disorders, insomnia, hyperemotivity and behaviour disorders. Otoneurologic examination is relevant in the identification and topographic diagnosis of vestibular disorders This chapter will verse on symptoms, audiometric and vestibular findings in TLC, as well as rehabilitation perspectives.

Keywords: labyrinth concussion, head injury, vertigo, hearing loss, dizziness

1. Introduction

Head injuries, from mild to severe, with or without cranial or petrosal fractures, may lead to traumatic labyrinth concussion (also referred to as labyrinth commotion) (TLC) – a vestibular disorder comprising auditory, vestibular and neurovegetative symptoms which may last up to weeks or months.

TLC may be concomitant to central nervous system (CNS) injury (diffuse axonal injury in brainstem/cerebellum, post-traumatic vestibular migraine, post-concussion syndrome) [1, 2] with autonomic signs, such as tachycardia, headache, thermoregulatory instability, mydriasis, as well as memory loss, behavioural changes, emotional lability, executive dysfunction, and gait disorders.

Otoneurologic evaluation is paramount in the identification and diagnosis of vestibular disorders.

This chapter will verse on symptoms, audiometric and vestibular findings in TLC, as well as rehabilitation and treatment perspectives.

2. Historical considerations

The most recent definition of Traumatic Labyrinth Commotion is that of an auditory or vestibular dysfunction in the absence of a temporal bone fracture (TBF) [3], still, its causes remain poorly understood. For a long time, post-traumatic vestibular symptoms were regarded as psychogenic, which explains the lack of established evaluation protocols and rehabilitation perspectives [4, 5].

Several pathologists have searched the correct definition and cause of traumatic labyrinth commotion, one of the first being Samuel Moos, in 1871 Prussia (nowadays, Germany) in a post-mortem assessment of a soldier who had suffered a glancing gunshot wound to his left mastoid, developing consequent hearing loss, due to a labyrinth haemorrhage; other reported possible mechanisms are cochleovestibular nerve traction injury and the travelling pressure wave theory, causing ciliary loss and cochlear damage [3].

Another possible clinical presentation is benign paroxysmal positional vertigo (BPPV) owed to dislodgement of otoconia from the macula of the utricle due to trauma, which should always be considered in patients with positional vertigo complaint after traumatic injuries, as well as utriculo-sacular injuries [2].

Romero characterised TLC as a disturbance of the inner ear with no evidence of macroscopic or radiological lesions, associated or not to central nervous system ailments, manifesting with vertigo, hypoacusis and tinnitus [6].

Also, there was a time in which it was believed labyrinth commotion was only related to head trauma severe enough to cause loss of conscience; yet, evidence has shown mild to moderate blunt trauma might lead to permanent neurosensorial hearing loss, compromising frequencies from 3.000 to 8000 Hz [7] or 4000 to 8000 Hz [8], as seen in noise-induced hearing loss [9, 10].

In 1976, TLC was regarded by Ganança and cols. as a peripheral syndrome, with the intensity of symptoms depending on the severity of the trauma, and that labyrinth areflexia was associated with mastoidal fracture, even when radiological evidence might have been absent, and traumatic facial palsy would be commonly found, often needing surgical correction [11].

This presentation is common in the context of commotions in the occipital region, leading to transversal temporal bone fractures (20%) or parietal/temporal commotions, leading to longitudinal fractures (80%). In transversal fractures, vestibular impairment tends to be unilateral; but may be bilateral, due to countercoup mechanism; in longitudinal fractures, anatomical damage usually comprises middle ear structures, with hearing loss, and vestibular symptomatology as a result of commotion of the membranous labyrinth [12, 13].

In Berman and cols' sample, most patients with vertigo after head trauma presented with post-concussion syndrome (PCS): headache, irritability, memory loss, autonomic symptoms, vertigo, hyperacusis, fatigue, vision changes, disturbances in balance, confusion, dizziness, insomnia, neuropsychiatric symptoms and difficulty with concentration [1, 14].

The ICD-10 defines PCS symptoms above persisting longer than 3 weeks, although most patients recover in the first 7 to 10 days following an injury [14]. Post-concussion syndrome pathophysiology includes metabolic, autonomic nervous system damage, and microstructural injuries to the brain, leading to structural and microbiological changes, resulting even in increased atrophy and regional volume loss, in several cases [15].

Vertigo, in this context, might have been related to PCS, to TLC alone, to perilymphatic fistulae (with/without need of posterior surgical intervention) or to psychological factors (due to or worsened by these) [1, 16].

Jerger & Jerger observed sudden onset of hearing loss, fluctuating over the first 3 weeks to 6 months, with the persistence of acute frequencies impairment, albeit recovery of hearing thresholds to normal levels [9].

Type of hearing loss – neurosensorial, conductive or mixed – depended on the mechanism of trauma, as well as lateralization – unilateral or bilateral [9]; tinnitus may last throughout the first three or four months or become permanent [17].

Word recognition performance varied as well: cochlear lesions result in proportional impairment considering pure-tone audiometry and word recognition, while in retro cochlear lesions, word recognition is worsened disproportionally to hearing loss. In pure central auditory system disturbances, pure-tone audiometry and word recognition may be normal [9].

Acoustic immittance is undisturbed in cochlear and retro cochlear insults and altered in middle ear disorders [9].

Considering electronystagmography, central [10] and peripheral [18–20] patterns may be present. Positional nystagmus may be temporary, according to [21], and may disappear a year following trauma; De Clercq described a post-traumatic alternating nystagmus lasting for years [22].

3. Personal data and discussion

A study conducted by the author analysed fifty cases of traumatic labyrinth commotion due to multiple causes.

Individuals underwent comprehensive anamnesis, otorhinolaryngological exam (to discard other ear, nose and throat affections which could be confounding factors), as well as audiological and vestibular assessment. Audiological evaluation consisted of pure-tone audiometry, word recognition testing and acoustic immittance. Vestibular assessment comprised static and dynamic balance testing – through Romberg, Romberg-Barré and Unterberger testing as well as gait evaluation – and vectonystagmography.

Positional stationary nystagmus was evaluated as present (including vertigo complaint) or not present, as it follows: supine, right-ear down, left-ear-down, supine and with head tilted down 30°, and seated [23].

Spontaneous nystagmus was assessed at the frontal plane, with open and closed eyes, and semi-spontaneous nystagmus with a 30° deviation towards right and left, upwards and downwards.

Vectonystagmography was developed using BERGER – VN 106/3, with three register channels. Skin was cleaned using an alcoholic solution; on each patient, an electrode was placed using an electrolyte paste for fixation on the lateral angle of each eye and on the frontal midline, forming an isosceles triangle, which made it possible to check horizontal, vertical, and oblique eye movements, providing precise measurements of the slow component angular velocity of nystagmus.

Calibration was made using the biological calibrator BERGER CB 115 and regularity of tracings was assessed to enable comparisons between studies. In testing of spontaneous nystagmus and semispontaneous nystagmus the presence, direction, inhibiting effect of ocular fixation (IEOF) and the maximum slow component angular velocity (SCAV) of nystagmus were assessed.

A BERGER TB-1131 visual stimulator was used for horizontal optokinetic nystagmus evaluation, concerning presence, direction, maximum SCAV with clockwise and anticlockwise movement of the light source and the preponderant direction of nystagmus was calculated. Pendular tracking evaluated the presence and type of curve.

A ROVER BR-3201 rotating descending pendular chair was used to investigate pre- and post-rotatory nystagmus by the pendular swing rotatory test with stimulation of the anterior, lateral and posterior semi-circular canals: presence, direction, frequency after anticlockwise and clockwise rotation and calculation of the preponderant direction were done.

A BERGER OC-114 water otocalorimeter was used with water temperatures of 44°C and 30°C for caloric testing with the patient's head and trunk tilted backwards by 60° for adequate stimulation of the lateral semi-circular canals. Stimulation time for each ear was 40 sec per ear at each temperature (44°C and 30°C) and responses were recorded with eyes closed and after with eyes open to observe IEOF. The direction, absolute values of SCAV and calculation of the preponderant direction and labyrinthic predominance of post-caloric nystagmus.

Anamnesis found vertigo and dizziness as the principal vestibular complaints, tinnitus (26%) as the main auditory complaint, followed by hyperacusis (20%) and hypoacusis (18%). Additional symptomatic findings are in **Table 1** in Appendix A.

As to audiological findings, 76% had normal results and 24% had neurosensorial hearing loss; 96% had unaltered word recognition and 90% had unremarkable acoustic immittance (**Table 2** in Appendix A).

Regarding vestibular findings, the totality of individuals had normal static and dynamic balance testing, normal oculomotor calibration, and absence of spontaneous and semi-spontaneous nystagmus with eyes open; 14 (28%) had positional vertigo, 3 (6%) had positional nystagmus and 13 (26%) had closed eyes spontaneous nystagmus with SCAV over 10°/s. One case (2%) had per-rotatory nystagmus areflexia (**Table 3** in Appendix A).

Symptomatologic findings were consistent with previously reported data [1, 6, 9] and more recent evidence [13, 24–26].

Normal auditory function seemed to be expected [17, 21], although Griffiths, in 1979, reported an incidence of 56% of hearing loss in his sample [27]. When present, neurosensorial hearing loss was the most prevalent, consistent with findings of numerous studies in the field [7, 9, 10, 16, 27, 28].

In our sample, vestibular findings were consistent with a peripheral deficit syndrome, as Mangabeira, Albernaz & Ganança [18] and conflicting with Kirtane's study, which found a higher incidence of central lesions, with absence of inhibitor effect of ocular fixation and enhanced caloric responses [10]. This might be due to different mechanisms of trauma and possible brainstem/central nervous system involvement, rather than pure TLC, in their sample, given that more recent studies have supported the fact that pure labyrinth commotion is a peripheral disorder, either by damage of the inner ear or of the vestibular nerve/apparatus [1, 13, 29].

Closed eyes spontaneous nystagmus with SCAV higher than 10°/s was reported in other studies [1, 22], as well as reduced caloric responses [1, 22].

The importance of a full otoneurologic evaluation in the context of post-concussion patients was once more reasserted, as the patients might present with unremarkable evidence of balance disorders at physical examination, and, yet, their exams might be abnormal, as postulated by Haid and Graeffe [19].

4. Rehabilitation and treatment perspectives

Treatment should be tailored according to patient individual necessities, severity, and mechanism of trauma, assessed thoroughly by a comprehensive and integrated approach, involving doctors, physiotherapists, speech therapists/audiologists, psychotherapists, and patients' families [4, 5, 26].

There is no definitive treatment for labyrinth concussion [30], as physiopathology is varied, therefore rehabilitation and treatment must be based on the patient complaint.

The first, and perhaps most important step is validation. Most patients who experience head trauma have subjective and sometimes hard-to-define complaints (take dizziness, for instance), not always well measured by objective tests, which for years led to the belief that those could be of a psychogenic nature, delaying the establishment of treatment protocols, even though of now it is known treatment should be initiated as early as possible, to mitigate pathophysiological chains involved [4, 5].

Patients with chronic vertigo are prone to work absenteeism [2], and, if present, psychiatric comorbidities are associated with poorer responses to treatment [27, 31, 32].

Screening tools, such as a full neurological and physiotherapic examination, as well as imaging examinations, must be used to identify the main mechanism of vertigo/dizziness, to provide specific therapeutic – if peripheral, vestibular rehabilitation may be useful; if cerebellar or due to disruptions on cerebellar pathways, coordination training should be proposed; if due to vision sequelae, vision directed therapy is indicated; if due to proprioceptive impairment, proprioception training might be appropriate; and if orthopaedic lesions are involved, specific treatment must be carried out [12, 14].

Neurotransmitters involved in vertigo pathophysiology are fundamentally Glutamate, acetylcholine and gamma-aminobutyric acid (GABA). Glutamate mediates synaptic transmission, mainly through amino-3-hydroxy-5-methylisoxazole-4-proprionic acid (AMPA)–type glutamate receptors and maintains resting discharge potential and long-term modulation of stimuli through N-methyl-D-aspartate (NMDA)– type glutamate receptors. Acetylcholine appears to play an excitatory role in the vestibular nuclei and might be involved in vestibular compensation. GABA, as in other CNS structures, acts as an inhibitory neurotransmitter, as well as glycine. Noradrenaline, dopamine, serotonin and histamine are involved with less clear effects, working as modulators, especially regarding emesis [33].

Thus, pharmacological treatment of vertigo includes vestibular suppressant drugs, such as benzodiazepines, antihistamines, and anticholinergic agents, as well as calcium-channel antagonists (less used nowadays due to their known relation with drug-induced parkinsonism) [34, 35] and dopamine receptor antagonists. Although useful in the reduction of symptom intensity in the acute phase [33], their efficacy is little in post-concussion vertigo, and their use should be brief (maximum 3 weeks). Benzodiazepines may be particularly beneficial in co-morbidity with anxiety and depression, although should be briefly used, given they might lead to dependency [33]. Suggestions of use can be found in **Table 4**.

In mild brain trauma, there are studies investigating the use of amantadine, yet the results are preliminary [5].

If despite optimised pharmacological treatment and rehabilitation, vertigo persists, in case of lesions confined to the labyrinth, labyrinthectomy or vestibular nerve section might an option [36].

Hearing loss may be present and should be identified and treated, with hearing aids proper adapting, led by an experienced team of audiologists, and, in severe cases of labyrinth commotion, cochlear implantation may be required [37].

In rehabilitation of PCS, reassurance remains the major treatment, as most symptoms tend to resolve within 3 months; when headache is a main issue, medications such as amitriptyline [38], greater occipital nervous blocks [39], propranolol and indomethacin [40, 41] may be useful, depending on the characterisation of pain – as

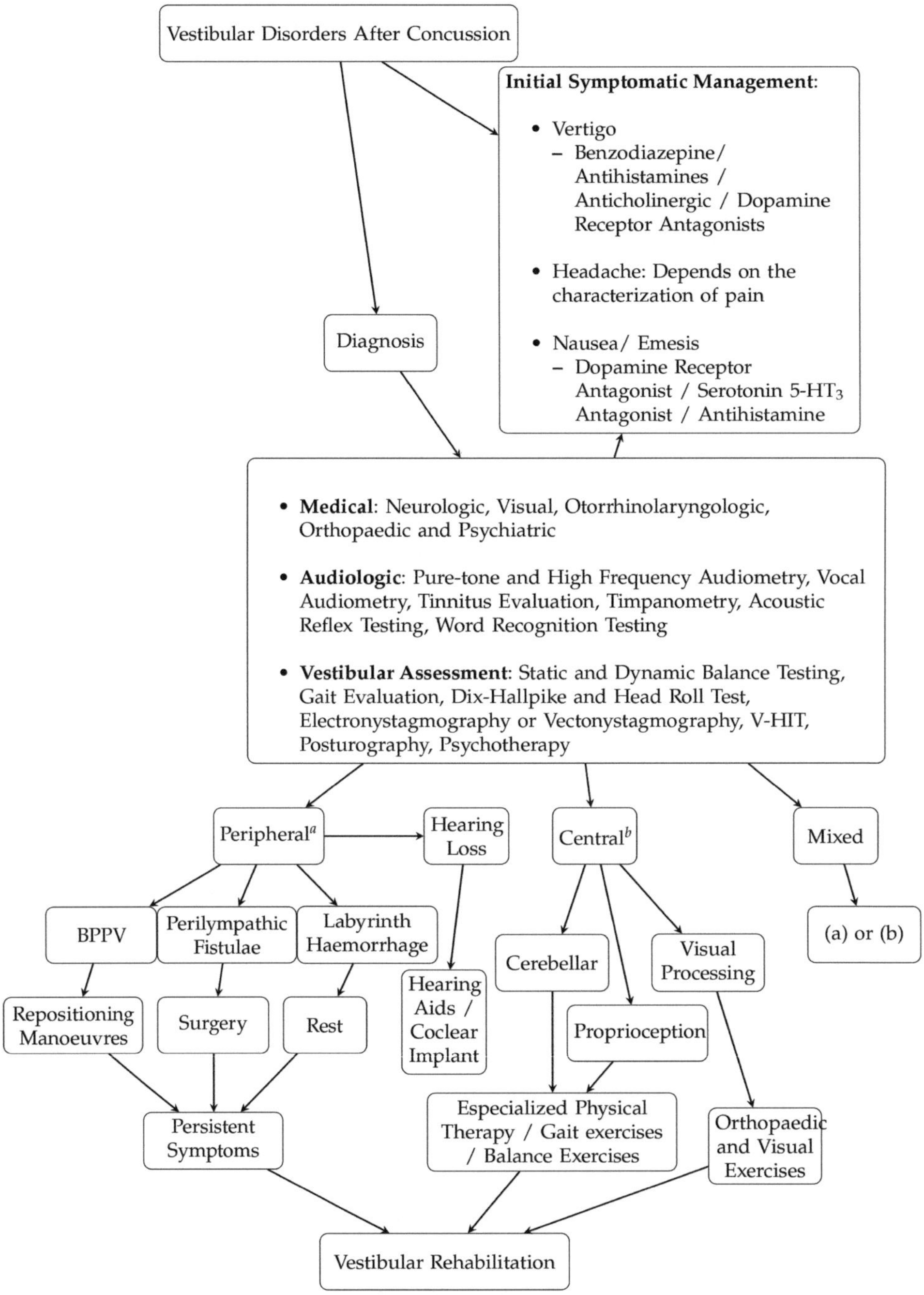

Figure 1.
Vestibular disorder management after head trauma.

post-concussive headaches often mimicry primary headaches, such as migraine, hemicrania continua and paroxysmal hemicrania.

Even patients with PCS may develop chronic vertigo or dizziness, chronic balance problems, or chronic cognitive impairment, which should also be assessed and treated.

Balance stability is one of the most multi-layered subjects in the field, given the complexity that underlies the mechanism of posture and gait control, comprising higher level processing, sensorial cues, proprioception, coordination, tone, strength, vestibular and visual cues [42]. Disruption in any of these points – neurologic, orthopaedic, psychologic, ophthalmologic, or audiologic – produces postural instability and, consequently, gait disturbances [43].

As such, the perfect balance rehabilitation should be able to evaluate all these fields, hence why a rehabilitation team is required. Posturography, kinematic evaluation, and sensorial integration in balance clinical testing are tools in the identification of the predominant deficiencies and help guide and plan therapy [12].

Otoneurologic assessment is not usually performed in the initial or follow-up of post-concussion patients [44, 45], although, as explained above, it might have benefit, including treatment planning.

A review by Nagib & Linens has brought evidence that vestibular rehabilitation (VRT), associated with light aerobic exercise or cervical spine therapy reduced Dizziness Handicap Index scores, improving quality of life and balance [46], whereas a study by Murray, Meldrum and Lennon also suggests that VRT might be useful in mild brain trauma, although more studies are necessary to fully establishment of the practice [47]. This evidence was also supported by the study of Park, Ksiazek and Olson, on VRT in adolescents who suffered sports-related concussion [25].

Wearable sensors and applications, if available, may be helpful in screening of brain injury extent through biomarkers [48], as well as monitoring physiological [49, 50], biological and gait data [51], to improve rehabilitation techniques, and prevent new trauma, as with fall detectors, detections of epileptic seizures and arrhythmias, as well as evaluate treatment efficacy [52]. Virtual and augmented reality systems have been also studied in the rehabilitation field, with promising results [53, 54], as well as audio-feedback [55].

Physical activity and aerobic exercise should always be encouraged, initially supervised, and, once the patient regains independence, unsupervised, as it correlates with autonomic regulation [24] cognitive recovery, by supporting neuroplasticity during the post-acute period [56], and re-establishing hippocampal homeostasis [57], due to activation of neuroprotective and antiapoptotic pathways, as well as mediating release of substances by bone, liver and muscle, augmenting brain production of brain-derived neurotrophic factor signalling (BDNF) [58–60], as well as improving quality of life and decreasing levels of anxiety, depression and permanent post-concussive symptoms [61–63] (**Figure 1**).

5. Concluding remarks

Traumatic Labyrinth Commotion may present with various otoneurological symptoms and signs, predominating vestibular over auditory alterations. Otoneurologic, audiological, neurological, and physical evaluations as well as image screening are relevant to treatment, which should be individualised and may comprise non-pharmacological, pharmacological and sometimes surgical interventions. It is suggested that vestibular rehabilitation may be useful in peripheral and central causes of vertigo and dizziness, as well as physical exercise may be an ally on rehabilitation of post-concussed patients.

Abbreviations

TLC	Traumatic Labyrinth Concussion
CNS	Central Nervous System
TBF	Temporal Bone Fracture
PCS	Post-Concussion Syndrome
ICD-10	International Classification of Diseases 2010
IEOF	Inhibiting Effect of Ocular Fixation
SCAV	slow component angular velocity
BNDF	Brain Derived Neutrophic Factor
AMPA	amino-3-hydroxy-5-methylisoxazole-4-proprionic acid
NMDA	N-methyl-D-aspartate
GABA	Gamma-aminobutyric Acid
VRT	Vestibular Rehabilitation Therapy
BPPV	Benign Paroxysmal Positional Vertigo

A. Appendix

Symptom	**No of cases**	**(%)**
Vertigo	32	64.0%
Dizziness	24	48.0%
Tinnitus	13	26.0%
Headache	11	22.0%
Hyperacusis	10	20.0%
Nausea	9	18.0%
Hypoacusis	9	18.0%
Ear pressure/fullness	8	16.0%
Sweating	7	14.0%
Phobias	7	14.0%
Pallor	6	12.0%
Depression	6	12.0%
Tachycardia	5	10.0%
Anxiety	5	10.0%
Sensation of "turning off"	4	8.0%
Darkening of vision	3	6.0%
Memory loss	3	6.0%
Falls	2	4.0%

Symptom	No of cases	(%)
Light-headedness	2	4.0%
Sleep disorders	2	4.0%
Vomiting	1	2.0%
Word recognition problems	1	2.0%
Feeling of liquid inside ear	1	2.0%
Ear pain	1	2.0%
Diplacusis	0	0

Table 1.
Prevalence of symptoms in 50 cases of traumatic labyrinth concussion.

Audiological findings	N° of cases	(%)
Tonal audiometry		
Normal	38	76.0%
Neuro-sensorial hearing loss	12	24.0%
Conductive hearing loss	0	0
Mixed hearing loss	0	0
Word recognition testing		
Normal	48	96.0%
Altered	2	4.0%
Acoustic immittance testing		
Normal	45	90.0%
Altered	5	10.0%

Table 2.
Prevalence of audiological findings in 50 cases of traumatic labyrinth concussion.

Vestibular findings	No. of cases	(%)
Normal balance (static and dynamic)	50	100.0%
Regular eye movement calibration	50	100.0%
Symmetric optokinetic nystagmus	50	100.0%
Pendular tracking types I or II	50	100.0%
Symmetric per-rotatory nystagmus	37	74.0%
Symmetric post-caloric nystagmus	24	48.0%
Positional vertigo	14	28.0%
Post-caloric nystagmus directional preponderance	14	28.0%
Spontaneous nystagmus with closed eyes (> 10°/s)	13	26.0%

Vestibular findings	No. of cases	(%)
Directional preponderance of per-rotatory nystagmus to lateral semi-circular channels stimulation	13	26.0%
Post-caloric nystagmus unilateral hyporeflexia	9	18.0%
Directional preponderance of per-rotatory nystagmus to vertical semi-circular channels stimulation	4	8.0%
Positional nystagmus	3	6.0%
Bilateral post-caloric nystagmus hyporeflexia	2	4.0%
Per-rotatory nystagmus areflexia	1	2.0%
Unilateral post-caloric nystagmus areflexia	1	2.0%
Bilateral post-caloric nystagmus areflexia	0	0
Post-caloric unilateral nystagmus hyperreflexia	0	0
Post-caloric bilateral nystagmus hyperreflexia	0	0

Table 3.
Prevalence of vestibular findings in 50 cases of traumatic labyrinth concussion.

Medication	Dosage[a]	Class	Side Effects and Precautions
Meclizine	Oral tablets 12.5–50 mg every 4-6 h or chewable tablets 25 mg tid	Antihistamine, anticholinergic	Sedating, dry mouth, urinary retention, bradycardia, precaution in prostatic enlargement and glaucoma
Clonazepam	0.5 mg orally bid	Benzodiazepine	Mildly sedating, incoordination, hallucinations, drug dependency
Scopolamine	0.5 mg patch every 3 days	Anticholinergic	Topical allergy, dry mouth, bradycardia, urinary retention, precaution in glaucoma
Dimenhydrinate	50 mg orally, IM or IV every 4–6 h	Antihistamine, anticholinergic	Sedating, dry mouth, urinary retention, bradycardia, precaution in prostatic enlargement and glaucoma
Diazepam	2–10 mg (one dose) given acutely orally, IM or IV or 2 mg orally bid	Benzodiazepine	Sedating, respiratory depressant, drug dependency, contraindicated in closed angle glaucoma
Lorazepam	0.5 mg orally or IM bid	Benzodiazepine	Mildly sedating, incoordination, hallucinations,

Medication	Dosage[a]	Class	Side Effects and Precautions
			drug dependency, contraindicated in closed angle glaucoma
Metoclopramide	10 mg orally tid or 10 mg IM	Dopamine antagonist, stimulates, upper gastrointestinal motility	Restlessness or drowsiness, extrapyramidal reaction
Promethazine	25 mg orally every 6–8 h, 25 mg rectally every 12 h or 12.5 mg IM every 6–8 h	Antihistamine	Sedating, extrapyramidal reaction, contraindicated in closed-angle glaucoma
Ondansetron	4 mg orally or IV.	Serotonin 5-HT3 antagonist	Headache, diarrhoea, fever

[a]*Recommended dosage for adults. Bid = twice daily; IM = intramuscularly; IV = intravenously; tid = three times daily.*

Table 4.
Pharmacological options to mitigate vertigo.

Author details

Maria Cristina Alves Corazza[1*], Luíza Alves Corazza[2†] and Júlia Alves Corazza[3‡]

1 University of Western São Paulo - College of Medicine, Presidente Prudente, SP, Brazil

2 Santa Marcelina Hospital - Department of Neurology, São Paulo, SP, Brazil

3 Federal University of Mato Grosso do Sul - College of Computing, Campo Grande, MS, Brazil

*Address all correspondence to: criscorazza40@gmail.com

†These authors contributed equally.

‡Draft review and formatting.

References

[1] Berman J, Fredrickson J. Vertigo after head injury–a five year follow-up. The Journal of otolaryngology. 1978;**7**(3): 237-245. Available from: http://europe pmc.org/abstract/MED/151151

[2] Fife TD, Giza C. Posttraumatic vertigo and dizziness. In: Seminars in Neurology. Vol. 33. New York, NY: Thieme Medical Publishers; 2013. p. 238-243

[3] Bartholomew RA, Lubner RJ, Knoll RM, Ghanad I, Jung D, Nadol JB Jr, et al. Labyrinthine concussion: Historic otopathologic antecedents of a challenging diagnosis. Laryngoscope Investigative Otolaryngology. 2020;**5**(2):267-277

[4] Rytter HM, Graff HJ, Henriksen HK, Aaen N, Hartvigsen J, Hoegh M, et al. Nonpharmacological treatment of persistent postconcussion symptoms in adults: A systematic review and meta-analysis and guideline recommendation. JAMA Network Open. 2021;**4**(11): e2132221-e2132221

[5] Kim K, Priefer R. Evaluation of current post-concussion protocols. Biomedicine & Pharmacotherapy. 2020; **129**:110406

[6] Briceño R. Lecciones de otorrinolaringología. Caracas: Talleres de Artegrafía; 1971

[7] Merchant SN, Nadol JB, editors. Schuknecht's Pathology of the Ear. PMPH-USA; 2010

[8] Browning GG, Swan IR, Gatehouse S. Hearing loss in minor head injury. Archives of Otolaryngology. 1982; **108**(8):474-477

[9] Jerger S, Jerger J. Auditory Disorders: A Manual for Clinical Evaluation. Boston, MA: Little Brown and Company; 1981

[10] Kirtane MV, Medikeri SB, Karnik PP. E.N.G. after head injury. The Journal of Laryngology & Otology. 1982;**96**(6):521-528

[11] Mangabeira-Albernaz P, Ganança M, Pontes P, Mangabeira-Albernaz P, Ganança M. Modelo operacional do aparelho vestibular. Mangabeira-Albernaz PL, Ganança MM Vertigem. 1976;**2**:29-36

[12] Shumway-Cook A. Rehabilitation of Vestibular Dysfunction in Traumatic Brain Njury. Physical Medicine and Rehabilitation Clinics of North America. Traumatic Brain Injury. 1992;**3**(2):355-69. Available from: https://www.scie ncedirect.com/ science/article/pii/ S1047965118306508

[13] Alkathiry AA, Sparto PJ, Kontos AP, Furman JM. Vestibular dysfunction associated with mild traumatic brain injury (mTBI). In: Neurosensory Disorders in Mild Traumatic Brain Injury. Cambridge, MA: Academic Press, Elsevier; 2019. pp. 133-148

[14] Permenter CM, Fernández-de Thomas RJ, Al S. Postconcussive syndrome. In: StatPearls. Treasure Island (FL): StatPearls Publishing; 2022

[15] Zhou Y, Kierans A, Kenul D, Ge Y, Rath J, Reaume J, et al. Mild traumatic brain injury: Longitudinal regional brain volume changes. Radiology. 2013;**267**(3): 880-890

[16] Nelson JR. Neuro-otologic aspects of head injury. Advances in Neurology. 1979;**22**:107-128

[17] Rubin W, Busis S, Brookler K. Otoneurologic examination.

Otolaryngology Philadelphia: JB Lippincott Company. 1993;**1**(9):1-47

[18] Mangabeira Albernaz PL, Ganança MM, Caovilla HH, Ito YI, Novo NF, Juliano Y. Aspectos clínicos e terapeuticos das vertigens. Acta Awho. 1986;**5**(Suppl. 2):49-109

[19] Haid C, Graeff G. Vertigo, a frequent symptom following cranial injury. Proceedings of the Neuro-otologicaland Equilibriometric. Society Reg. 1983;**9**: 22-36

[20] Khalek A. Head injuries persistent post-concussion symptoms. The British Journal of Clinical Practice. 1983;**37**(6): 209-211

[21] El GV. oido enfermedades sordera y vértigo. 1st ed. Mallorca, Spain: Salvat; 1986

[22] De Clercq H, Naude A, Bornman J. Investigating nystagmus in patients with traumatic brain injury: A systematic review (1996-2016). South African Medical Journal. 2017;**107**(11): 957-964

[23] Mangabeira Albernaz P, Ganança M, Caovilla H, Ito Y, Castro H. Atlas de vecto-electronistagmografia. São Paulo: Aché; 1984

[24] Leddy JJ, Haider MN, Ellis M, Willer BS. Exercise is medicine for concussion. Current sports medicine reports. 2018;**17**(8):262

[25] Park K, Ksiazek T, Olson B. Effectiveness of vestibular rehabilitation therapy for treatment of concussed adolescents with persistent symptoms of dizziness and imbalance. Journal of sport rehabilitation. 2018;**27**(5):485-490

[26] Gurley JM, Hujsak BD, Kelly JL. Vestibular rehabilitation following mild traumatic brain injury. NeuroRehabilitation. 2013;**32**(3):519-528

[27] Griffiths MV. The incidence of auditory and vestibular concussion following minor head injury. The Journal of Laryngology and Otology. 1979;**93**(3): 253-265

[28] Vartiainen E, Karjalainen S, Kärjä J. Auditory disorders following head injury in children. Acta Oto-Laryngologica. 1985;**99**(5–6):529-536

[29] Chiaramonte R, Bonfiglio M, D'amore A, Viglianesi A, Cavallaro T, Chiaramonte I. Traumatic labyrinthine concussion in a patient with sensorineural hearing loss. The Neuroradiology Journal. 2013;**26**(1): 52-55

[30] Villarreal I, Méndez D, Silva J, Álamo P. Contralateral cochlear labyrinthine concussion without temporal bone fracture: Unusual posttraumatic consequence. Case reports in Otolaryngology. 2016;**2016**:1055-1058

[31] Jacobs GB, Lehrer JF, Rubin RC, Hubbard JH, Nalebuff DJ, Wille RL. Posttraumatic vertigo. Report of three cases. Journal of Neurosurgery. 1979; **51**(6):860-861

[32] Long C, Novack T. Postconcussion symptoms after head trauma: Interpretation and treatment. Southern Medical Journal. 1986;**79**(6):728-732

[33] Hain TC, Uddin M. Pharmacological treatment of vertigo. CNS Drugs. 2003; **17**(2):85-100

[34] Teive HA, Munhoz RP, Ferraz HB. Flunarizine and cinnarizine-induced parkinsonism: 25 years of de Melo-Souza's syndrome. Arquivos de Neuro-Psiquiatria. 2009;**67**:957-957

[35] Lin HL, Lin HC, Tseng YF, Chen SC, Hsu CY. Risk of parkinsonism induced by flunarizine or cinnarizine: A population-based study. European journal of clinical pharmacology. 2017; **73**(3):365-371

[36] Katz J, Chasin M, English KM, Hood LJ, Tillery KL. Handbook of Clinical Audiology. Vol. 7. PA: Wolters Kluwer Health Philadelphia; 2015

[37] Colucci D. Understanding labyrinthine concussion. The Hearing Journal. 2017;**70**(4):44-46

[38] Tyler GS, McNeely HE, Dick ML. Treatment of post-traumatic headache with amitriptyline. Headache: The Journal of Head and Face Pain. 1980; **20**(4):213-216

[39] Hecht JS. Occipital nerve blocks in postconcussive headaches: A retrospective review and report of ten patients. The Journal of head trauma rehabilitation. 2004;**19**(1):58-71

[40] Lay CL, Newman LC. Posttraumatic hemicrania continua. Headache: The Journal of Head and Face Pain. 1999; **39**(4):275-279

[41] Matharu MS, Goadsby PJ. Post-traumatic chronic paroxysmal hemicrania (CPH) with aura. Neurology. 2001;**56**(2):273-275

[42] Baker JM. Gait disorders. The American journal of medicine. 2018; **131**(6):602-607

[43] Akin FW, Murnane OD, Hall CD, Riska KM, Sears J. Vestibular and balance function in veterans with chronic dizziness associated with mild traumatic brain injury and blast exposure. Frontiers in Neurology. 2022; **13**:930389

[44] Scorza KA, Cole W. Current concepts in concussion: Initial evaluation and management. American Family Physician. 2019;**99**(7):426-434

[45] Silverberg ND, Iaccarino MA, Panenka WJ, Iverson GL, McCulloch KL, Dams-O'Connor K, et al. Management of concussion and mild traumatic brain injury: A synthesis of practice guidelines. Archives of Physical Medicine and Rehabilitation. 2020;**101**(2):382-393

[46] Nagib S, Linens SW. Vestibular rehabilitation therapy improves perceived disability associated with dizziness postconcussion. Journal of Sport Rehabilitation. 2019;**28**(7): 764-768

[47] Murray DA, Meldrum D, Lennon O. Can vestibular rehabilitation exercises help patients with concussion? A systematic review of efficacy, prescription and progression patterns. British Journal of Sports Medicine. 2017; **51**(5):442-451

[48] Schmid W, Fan Y, Chi T, Golanov E, Regnier-Golanov AS, Austerman RJ, et al. Review of wearable technologies and machine learning methodologies for systematic detection of mild traumatic brain injuries. Journal of Neural Engineering. 2021;**18**(4):041006

[49] Adans-Dester C, Hankov N, O'Brien A, Vergara-Diaz G, Black-Schaffer R, Zafonte R, et al. Enabling precision rehabilitation interventions using wearable sensors and machine learning to track motor recovery. NPJ Digital Medicine. 2020;**3**:121

[50] Stuart S, Parrington L, Martini D, Kreter N, Chesnutt J, Fino P, et al. Analysis of free-living mobility in people with mild traumatic brain injury and healthy controls: Quality over quantity. Central Nervous System Trauma. 2020;

37(1):139-145. Funding Information: This work was supported by the Assistant Secretary of Defense for Health Affairs under Award No. W81XWH-15-1-0620. Opinions, interpretations, conclusions and recommendations are those of the author and are not necessarily endorsed by the Department of Defense. Publisher Copyright: © Copyright 2020, Mary Ann Liebert, Inc., publishers

[51] Belluscio V, Bergamini E, Tramontano M, Orejel Bustos A, Allevi G, Formisano R, et al. Gait quality assessment in survivors from severe traumatic brain injury: An instrumented approach based on inertial sensors. Sensors. 2019;**19**(23):5315

[52] Patel S, Park H, Bonato P, Chan L, Rodgers M. A review of wearable sensors and systems with application in rehabilitation. Journal of Neuroengineering and Rehabilitation. 2012;**9**(1):1-17

[53] Rodgers MM, Alon G, Pai VM, Conroy RS. Wearable technologies for active living and rehabilitation: Current research challenges and future opportunities. Journal of rehabilitation and assistive technologies engineering. 2019;**6**:2055668319839607

[54] Grealy MA, Johnson DA, Rushton SK. Improving cognitive function after brain injury: The use of exercise and virtual reality. Archives of Physical Medicine and Rehabilitation. 1999;**80**(6):661-667. Available from: https://www.sciencedirect.com/science/article/pii/S0003999399901697

[55] Campbell K, Peterka R, Fino P, Parrington L, Wilhelm J, Pettigrew N, et al. The effects of augmenting traditional rehabilitation with audio biofeedback in people with persistent imbalance following mild traumatic brain injury. Frontiers in Neurology. 2022;**13**:926691

[56] Kreber LA, Griesbach GS. The interplay between neuropathology and activity based rehabilitation after traumatic brain injury. Brain Research. 2016;**1640**:152-163

[57] Archer T. Influence of physical exercise on traumatic brain injury deficits: Scaffolding effect. Neurotoxicity Research. 2012;**21**(4):418-434

[58] Stephan JS, Sleiman SF. Exercise factors as potential mediators of cognitive rehabilitation following traumatic brain injury. Current Opinion in Neurology. 2019;**32**(6):808-814. Available from:. DOI: 10.1097/WCO.0000000000000754

[59] Morris T, Gomes Osman J, Tormos Muñoz JM, Costa Miserachs D, Pascual LA. The role of physical exercise in cognitive recovery after traumatic brain injury: A systematic review. Restorative Neurology and Neuroscience. 2016;**34**(6):977-988. Available from:. DOI: 10.3233/RNN-160687

[60] Zhao Z, Sabirzhanov B, Wu J, Faden AI, Stoica BA. Voluntary exercise preconditioning activates multiple Antiapoptotic mechanisms and improves neurological recovery after experimental traumatic brain injury. Journal of Neurotrauma. 2015;**32**(17):1347-1360

[61] Wise EK, Hoffman JM, Powell JM, Bombardier CH, Bell KR. Benefits of exercise maintenance after traumatic brain injury. Archives of Physical Medicine and Rehabilitation. 2012;**93**(8):1319-1323. Available from: https://www.sciencedirect.com/science/article/pii/S0003999312003541

[62] Chin LMK, Keyser RE, Dsurney J, Chan L. Improved cognitive performance following aerobic exercise training in people with traumatic brain injury. Archives of Physical Medicine and Rehabilitation. 2015;**96**(4):754-759

[63] Haider MN, Bezherano I, Wertheimer A, Siddiqui AH, Horn EC, Willer BS, et al. Exercise for sport-related concussion and persistent postconcussive symptoms. Sports Health. 2021;**13**(2):154-160

Chapter 6

A Similarity Index for Balance Assessment between Older Adults with and without Balance Deficits

Paul S. Sung and Dongchul Lee

Abstract

Falls in older adults can cause disabling health even though falls are largely preventable. A combination of fall risk factors can be modified or predicted to minimize devastating complications. However, clinical balance assessment tools often have contradictory results since fall risks are individualized and multifactorial. The assessment tools are often practically limited to detecting sensitive changes between older adults with and without balance deficits. Recently, a similarity index (SI) has been developed to predict fall risks based on kinematic data during gait. The combined limb motions to those of a prototype derived from healthy individuals in the gait cycle might be differentiated from individuals with gait pathologies. The analyzed calculations result in response vectors that would be compared to controls-derived prototype response vectors. Furthermore, the normalized SI, based on the vector representing the data distribution, could be generated from the enhanced (dis)similarities dataset of subjects following an intervention (prototype response vectors). These quantified indices for compensatory patterns provide a further understanding of optimal injury prevention and specific rehabilitation strategies for older adults with balance deficits. This chapter will propose a novel sensitive measure, the SI, for older adults with orthopedic and neurologic dysfunction compared with control subjects.

Keywords: kinematic, similarity index, balance deficits, pain, older adults, gait cycle, motions

1. Introduction

Balance problems in older adults are of major concern as functional declines of the somatosensory system occur in aging populations, potentially contributing to postural instability [1, 2]. These problems provide foundational knowledge of balance performance and the importance of using a reliable and valid sensory testing protocol for older adults. However, valid balance measurements are burdensome and costly, especially for older adults with balance deficits who are characterized by greater comorbidity compared to healthy adults [3]. As a result, it would be critical to evaluate the characteristics of falls and clarify the advantages of predicting the occurrence of falls in older adults with balance deficits.

Previous studies utilized clinical measure tools, such as the Berg Balance Scale (BBS), the Dynamic Gait Index (DGI), as well as other advanced balance measures [4–6]. However, the small sample size in their studies limits the validity of the results to generalize measurement outcomes. A sensitive balance detection tool with a larger sample size can be compared to examine balance deficits. It would be valuable to utilize a valid tool based on both scientific understanding and clinical applications of balance mechanisms in older adults. Previous research reports did not necessarily prove the sensitive outcome assessment by detailing how the feasibility of those measurement tools will achieve fall assessment and prevention. However, our studies attempted to comprehensively evaluate outcomes by introducing biomechanical research and clinical applications on biomechanics and neuromuscular control during functional activities [7–9].

A similarity index (SI) tool provides a detailed picture of different limb and trunk muscle activations by electromyography (EMG) and kinematic stability during gait. Most older adults with balance deficits present with impaired postural control [10–12] and motor coordination, including the inability to initiate, continue, or terminate activation of multiple muscle groups in a task- and environment-specific manner [13, 14]. However, the existing balance assessment tools often lack clinical evidence and demonstrate conflicting outcomes. It is critical to compare age- and gender-matched groups with balance deficits using clinical measurement tools. These tests evaluate dynamic stability in older adults with balance deficits related to somatosensory impairments in musculoskeletal and neurologic symptoms.

2. Gait assessment in individuals with musculoskeletal dysfunction

Decreased physical activity levels result in a concomitant decline in musculoskeletal function. Adequate muscular strength is fundamental to preserving functional mobility from asymmetrical limb motions during gait, which has been an increasingly important theme of research in recent years [15–17]. These studies predicted the risk of falls from the gait measures, and there is an increased risk of multiple falls in older adults with poor gait. Specific measures of gait and gait variability from musculoskeletal dysfunction confer the balance deficits and could be amenable to reducing the risk of falls.

Neck dysfunction/pain is the fourth leading cause of disability and the most common musculoskeletal disorder in primary care [18, 19]. Several studies reported that individuals with neck pain have impairments of balance and head-neck coordination as well as sensorimotor deficits including poorer proprioception [20–22]. However, there is a lack of understanding of gait parameters and the kinematic SI on the limbs during gait. The similarity of gait patterns and compensated limb motions in individuals with neck pain compared to healthy controls was not carefully investigated. If the similarity of the combined limb motions is lessened in individuals with neck pain compared with healthy controls, then those kinematic changes might be detected in the specific phases of the gait cycle. The magnitude of motions and the degree of similarity between groups may provide clinical insights to enhance a comprehensive understanding of the functional consequences of gait deviations.

A recent study indicated that SI was a useful measure to differentiate similarities between groups at specific phases during gait [23]. The kinematic SI during gait was investigated to compare the ratio between the vector representing the distribution of the motions in individuals with neck pain and that representing the average distribution in individuals without neck pain. These SI values of the control group were significantly higher than the neck pain group during gait, especially in the midstance and swing phases. The SI could have the potential to highlight differences in the neck pain group during gait more than common parameters, such as cadence, speed, stride length, and step width. Ultimately, an objective measure, such as the SI, may enhance gait evaluations and help to determine the similarity of combined kinematic changes during gait.

The SI measure could provide an objective tool for the overall kinematic variations and similarities that occur during gait between groups as well. For example, an altered gait pattern was evident in individuals with neck pain who demonstrated a slower and more asymmetrical gait [24]. Therefore, the similarities of the combined upper and lower limbs might clarify the difference in gait patterns between individuals with and without neck pain. It is valuable to identify the specific phases of gait and to compare the similarity between individuals with and without neck pain. The normalized SI measures were from three-dimensional (3D) motions and provide quantitative evidence at 5% intervals of the entire gait cycle. The collected data may guide design to improve gait function.

2.1 Methodology of the kinematic similarity index

Spatiotemporal and kinematic parameters were calculated for each gait cycle using OrthoTrac 5.2 software (Motion Analysis Corporation, Santa Rosa, CA, USA). The spatiotemporal parameters included cadence, gait speed, stride length, and step width. Three-dimensional upper and lower limb kinematic waveforms were time normalized to 100 points, comprising the gait cycle from 0 to 100% with 1% increments [25, 26].

The kinematic SI computation is a numerical expression of the motion similarity in the response vectors (RV) between participants with and without neck pain (NP). The SI was computed as the normalized cosine angle (θ), where θ is the angle between two vectors, which were prototype and response vectors. The prototype response vector (PRV) represented the distribution of activity generated by participants without neck pain (NP), and the response vector (RV) represented the distribution of the participants with neck pain (NP). The RV was a series of elements with angles of each joint at a specific time point during gait for each subject. The PRV was an average of response vectors from the control participants. The mathematical equation for computing SI, the cosine of the angle between two vectors, is indicated in Equation (1).

The kinematic data included the bilateral shoulders, elbows, hips, knees, and ankles. However, the elbow did not possess frontal or transverse motions, and the shoulder possessed negligible transverse motion during gait. To quantify the gait patterns, the SI was computed from kinematic data using Equation (1), which is the summation of the corresponding elements (numerator), divided by the magnitude of both vectors (denominator).

$$SI_x = \frac{\sum_i \left(PRV_{x_i} . RV_{x_i}\right)}{|PRV_x||RV_x|} \tag{1}$$

PRVx= [PRVx_1, PRVx_1, ... PRVx_n] at x% during gait. PRVx_1: averaged value of L-Shoulder flexion angles (S) from all control participants. PRVx_2: averaged value of L-Shoulder abduction angles (F) from all control participants. PRVx_n: averaged value of n'th channel from all control participants. RVx= [RVx_1, RVx_2, ... RVx_n] at x% during gait. RVx_1: L-Shoulder flexion angles (S) from a participant with NP. RVx_2: L-Shoulder abduction angles (F) from a participant with NP. RVx_n: n'th channel from a participant with NP.

The element of this vector is the angle of joints in the 3D directions at increments of 5% in the gait cycle, and the SI is constrained to be between 0 and 1. A normalized SI value of 1.0 designates an angle of zero between two vectors (i.e., the RV had an identical distribution to PRV) and signifies that motions in participants with neck pain are identical to that of the population. In **Figure 1**, the RVx is the vector with elements of individual joint angles at a specific point in the gait cycle (x%). The SI_x was computed by comparison between PRV_x and RV_x and as the cosine of angles between the two vectors. To cover the full gait cycle (0 to 100%), PRV_x and RV_x were computed at increments of 5% in the gait cycle. The SI equation was formulated between the participants with and without neck pain (where i represents 3D kinematic data/channel, and x represents the gait cycle out of 100%). Previous studies reported the mathematical description and an example of the computation of the index [27–30]. To compute a time-variant SI during gait, PRVs and RVs were computed at 5% increments of the entire gait cycle and compared between PRV and RV from corresponding segments. Therefore, the kinematic SI is a quantitative measurement of how similar a given RV is to the PRV.

As shown in **Figure 2**, the results of the study indicated that the neck pain group demonstrated a greater variation of walking patterns during the midstance and swing phases and displayed altered compensatory gait. The SI values for the gait cycle were higher in the control group than the NP group (0.98 ± 0.02 vs. 0.95 ± 0.03). The standard deviation of the SI was significantly less in the control group compared to

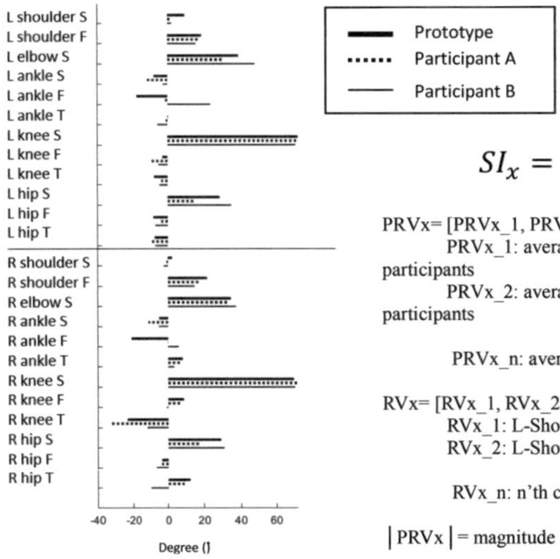

$$SI_x = \frac{\sum_i (PRV_{x\_i} \cdot RV_{x\_i})}{|PRV_x||RV_x|} \quad \text{Eq. 1}$$

PRVx= [PRVx_1, PRVx_1, ... PRVx_n] at x% during gait

PRVx_1: averaged value of L-Shoulder flexion angles (S) from all control participants

PRVx_2: averaged value of L-Shoulder abduction angles (F) from all control participants

PRVx_n: averaged value of n'th channel from all control participants

RVx= [RVx_1, RVx_2, ... RVx_n] at x% during gait

RVx_1: L-Shoulder flexion angles (S) from a participant with NP

RVx_2: L-Shoulder abduction angles (F) from a participant with NP

RVx_n: n'th channel from a participant with NP

| PRVx | = magnitude of the PRVx vector

| RVx | = magnitude of the RVx vector

Figure 1.
Example of SI computation. The left column shows the range of motions of the limbs during gait. The dark lines represent the averages of the control participants. Participant A with NP demonstrated good matching with the prototype in certain joints (R knee S, but mismatched in R hip S), and participant B with NP showed the opposite direction in L ankle abduction. On the right panel, Eq. 1 explains the principle of computing the SI. The PRVx is a vector with elements of individual joint angles at specific gate cycles, which was multiplied by averaging all control participants. (NP: neck pain, R: right, L: left, S: sagittal plane, F: frontal plane, T: transverse plane with all 24 (12 for each side) channels).

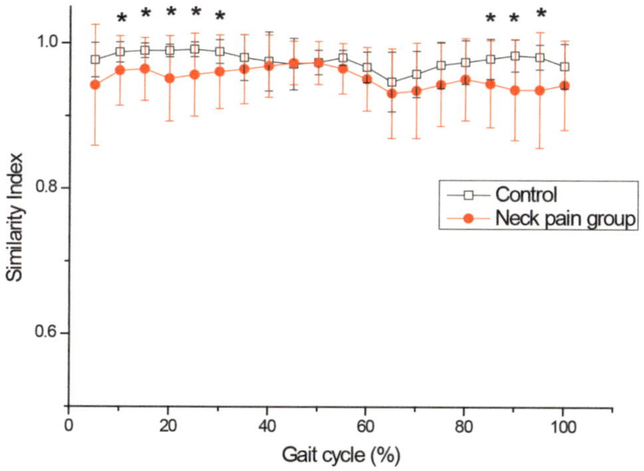

Figure 2.
The Similarity Index (SI) values were obtained from the control and neck pain groups at increments of 5% during the gait cycle. There were significant group differences at 10%, 15%, 20%, 25%, and 30% of the gait cycle in the midstance phase. In the terminal swing phase, the control group demonstrated significantly higher SI at 85%, 90%, and 95% of the gait cycle (< 0.05).*

the neck pain group (0.02 ± 0.01 vs. 0.04 ± 0.02). The similarities of the kinematic changes for the neck pain group were used to aid in the detection of limb motion differences and the resulting gait dysfunction. The SI values of the control group were significantly higher than the neck pain group during gait, especially at the midstance (10-30%) and swing (80-90%) phases. Also, the standard deviation of the SI decreased in the control group when compared to the neck pain group. The results were evident that the index reflects kinematic changes in limb functions during gait. There was less kinematic similarity in the neck pain group during gait due to a lack of similarities during the midstance and swing phases.

The neck pain group also demonstrated a greater standard deviation of the SI (ranges from 0.02 to 0.05 in the stance phase, ranges from 0.05 to 0.07 in the swing phase) compared to the control group, which was less than 0.02. The standard deviation of the SI was less in the control group compared to the neck pain group.

2.2 Clinical application of the kinematic similarity index

Although the gait parameters did not provide significant differences, the SI results detected gait deviations based on the kinematic data. The neck pain group may have modified their walking patterns, especially in the midstance and swing phases. Our results are warranted to investigate whole-body movement, including the trunk, for gait control, and early detection of gait deviations. Several studies reported that the SI provides sensitive measures as a neurophysiological method for characterizing voluntary motor control in human performance [27–31]. In our study, however, the SI concept was applied to kinematic data since the SI is a numerical expression of the similarity in distribution between participants with and without neck pain.

The importance of SI relies on the method that utilizes the kinematic data from every possible motion at a specific time point, while previous methods compared specific limb support patterns [32]. Therefore, the joint kinematic data based on the normal range (from PRV) can be detected by the SI computation. The SI concept is applicable to analyze the normalized kinematic data within and between groups for combined motions of the upper and lower limbs [27, 29], rather than for only a single joint motion in the gait cycle. Therefore, the SI is an important contribution to objective evaluations of the musculoskeletal system that could also be used to detect gait deviations.

Although our study was not intended to investigate the specific reasons for the differences, previous studies reported that the NP group could display biomechanical disturbances even with relatively mild pain and demonstrate reduced trunk rotation during gait, which indicates an increased stiffer spine [33, 34]. Previous studies were limited to clinical applications for gait dysfunction, since the distribution of the motions may provide a limited interpretation [32, 35]. A possible mechanism related to altered postural control during walking may be the consequence of diminished proprioceptive inputs leading to compensatory strategies to avoid pain or injury in the NP group [36]. The single limb support in midstance involves a progression of the body over the foot and weight-bearing stability. It is the first sub-phase where the shank rotates forward over the supporting foot, creating the second rocker motion of the cycle [37]. During the terminal swing, the final advancement of the shank takes place, and the foot is positioned for initial contact for the next gait cycle. These specific phases during gait are critical in developing effective gait strategies; however, the NP group may adapt or modify their strategies to accommodate any differences.

The differences between the SI with the combined limb motions in the midstance and swing phases during gait might be utilized to compare gait dysfunction. For example, the neck pain group may display subtle changes in load sharing and reduced conjunct neck motions in the frontal and sagittal planes during cervical rotation [38], which results in increased motion variabilities and reduced smoothness of limb motions. Therefore, the kinematic SI might be utilized to detect functional outcomes for gait dysfunction and/or balance deficits. Furthermore, clinicians need to consider gait evaluations when comparing kinematic variations for those phases, which likely reflect adaptive behavior for postural control.

Increased kinematic similarities were evident in the control group. Optimal stability and mobility might prevent potential injuries with combined trunk and limb motions [39, 40]. The results of our study also confirmed that the standard deviations of the kinematic SI decreased in the control group (**Figure 2**). The PRV was constructed from a limited set of control participants. It could be expected that individual variations and other confounding factors may provide slightly different PRVs. The SI concept would be valuable in building a database to evaluate kinematic variations between groups with and without dysfunction. There are different movement strategies that can possibly be adjusted, and the SI method detects the difference in gait dysfunctions. Further in-depth analyses could be developed for clinically meaningful and detailed insights into gait dysfunction.

3. Gait assessment between control subjects and post-stroke subjects

For post-stroke individuals, paralysis and muscle weakness in the upper and lower limbs can lead to balance, mobility disorders and gait function. There are guidelines intended for clinicians to optimize rehabilitation outcomes for subjects with chronic stroke to improve walking speed and distance. It has been generally accepted that stroke commonly results in trunk impairments that are associated with decreased trunk coordination and limited trunk muscle strength [41]. However, the guidelines limited ambulatory function due to the lack of sensitive assessments, which may not apply to the specific phase of the gait cycle in post-stroke individuals. These problems ultimately lead to a limit in functional activities and/or gait. Thus, the need for evaluation and rehabilitation methods in gait dysfunction has been emphasized on sensitive measures.

Surface EMG assessment of voluntary motor control provides a clinical manifestation of gait performance. The evidence suggests that frequency-based analysis of EMG can be used to detect cortical motor control contribution [42]. Characteristically, individuals post-stroke demonstrate slow gait velocity with residual spatial and temporal asymmetry when compared to healthy subjects. The changes in muscle activity in individuals with stroke differed between the paretic and nonparetic sides, muscle type, and gait phase; walking performance was maintained despite being affected by neuromuscular fatigue. These clinical manifestations in gait post-stroke result from deficits in limb movement as well as impairments in the control of trunk mobility [43]. Decreased anteroposterior movements of the thorax were the main variable explaining the gait function. Although trunk training is an effective strategy for improving mobility after stroke, the implementation and generalizability of this treatment approach in a clinical setting are laborious and limited. Since postural muscle activation is an integral part of motor control, it is important to investigate the activation patterns of the trunk muscles as well.

Other studies supported that neuromuscular control of gait post-stroke can be affected by changes in the trunk as well as the lower limb muscle activity patterns [41, 43]. Their impairments often result in biomechanical changes during gait. Specifically, pelvic motions might be influenced by these impairments. Following a stroke, patients walk with increased mediolateral trunk sway and larger sagittal motion of the lower trunk. Although the rotation of the upper trunk increases, the trunk shows more in-phase coordination. Acceleration of the trunk diminishes while instability and asymmetry increase as there are less movements toward the paretic side. However, it is of great importance to differentiate between compensatory trunk movements and intrinsic trunk control deficits. In **Figure 3**, the EMG analyses in the gait cycle, as averaged within the control group, were represented with solid dark lines in the first column and are regarded as the average of all strides in each muscle.

3.1 Methodology of the similarity index in gait cycle

Since the post-stroke group was not expected to have the same stance-to-swing ratio as compared with the control group even at similar gait speeds, data was normalized to eliminate this timing discrepancy. In general, post-stroke hemiparetic gait is slow compared with healthy individuals with asymmetry in the spatiotemporal parameters such as step length, swing time, stance time, and double-leg support time. Stance and swing phases were analyzed separately and then adjusted to a ratio of 60:40 percent for a graphic presentation of the gait cycle. In addition, EMG magnitude was normalized using the mean amplitude from the walking trials in a procedure similar to that reported by Benoit and colleagues [44].

The SI computation is a numerical expression of the similarity of the distribution of EMG activity in the response vectors (RV) between individuals with pathology (in this case, stroke) and a healthy population. The SI is computed as the normalized inner product, or the cosine of the solid angle between the vector representing the distribution of activity generated by healthy subjects (prototype response vector: PRV), and that representing the distribution in the test subjects (RV). Thus, the SI is constrained to lie between 0 and 1. An SI value of 1.0 designates an angle of zero (i.e., the RV had

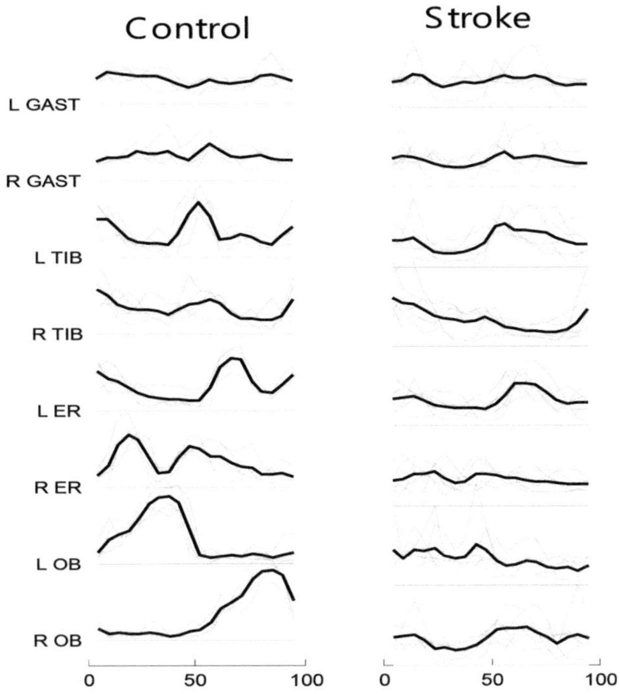

Figure 3.
EMG during gait cycle for control and stroke groups beginning at right foot contact (0%) to foot contact on the same side (100%). Individual control group EMG recordings, superimposed over the average with gray lines, demonstrated consistent patterns with small variability while individual EMG recordings for the stroke group had larger variability. This qualitative analysis of EMG patterns between the control and stroke groups suggests the spatial and temporal EMG distributions quantified by the SI. The control group demonstrated less variability than post-stroke individuals. Solid lines represent the average of all strides in each muscle from the group (EMG: electromyography, R: right, L: left, GAST: gastrocnemius, TIB: tibialis anterior, ER: erector spinae, OB: external oblique muscles).

an identical distribution of EMG activity to PRV) and signifies that muscle activity in pathological subjects is similar to that of a normal population.

The SI was computed only for RVs with a magnitude sufficient to differentiate a response from background noise. To compute a time-variant SI during the gait cycle, RVs were computed using a gait cycle segmented into 5% increments and compared to the PRVs from corresponding segments of the cycle. A gait cycle EMG, as averaged within the control group, is represented with solid dark lines in the first column of **Figure 1** and is regarded as the average of all strides in each muscle. Individual control group EMG recordings, superimposed over the average with gray lines, demonstrated consistent patterns with small variability while individual EMG recordings for the stroke group had larger variability. This qualitative analysis of EMG patterns between the control and stroke groups suggests the spatial and temporal EMG distributions quantified by the SI.

3.2 Clinical application of the similarity index during gait

This index explored the use of the SI as a method of quantifying changes in muscle activity as measured by EMG. Use of the SI indicated greater variation from the trunk muscles in normal subjects as compared to the lower limb muscles during gait in the post-stroke group. In addition, our results provided preliminary data related to trunk muscle activity in the lumbar erector spinae and the external oblique muscles, which is an area that has not been extensively reported during gait in the post-stroke group. According to the data from our lab, these differences in trunk muscle activity post-stroke peaked at 40% of the gait cycle, or 67% of the stance phase, and 90% of the gait cycle, or 75% of the swing phase. Trunk muscle activity post-stroke was most normal at 5% and 65% of the gait cycle, or 8% of the stance phase and 4% of the swing phase, which are the beginning portions of each phase.

In **Figure 4**, the SI values were obtained from the control and stroke groups without phase normalization for each 5% segment of the gait cycle. The mean of the SIs calculated for a whole gait cycle from the control group (0.965 ± 0.030) was higher than the post-stroke group (0.88 ± 0.077) when all muscles were used. The largest difference between the two groups was observed at 85-95% of the gait cycle, which would represent the middle of the swing phase if normal stance/swing phase durations were assumed. The post-stroke group showed much greater variability than the control group at all points in the cycle. The largest variability of the SI values in the post-stroke group was observed at 55% of the gait cycle. In the control group, the mean SI of each 5% segment throughout the entire gait cycle ranged from 0.965 to 0.968 with a variance of less than 0.20, which supports that the prototype represents the EMG patterns of the control group quite well.

Although the SI value from the total gait cycle for each of the two groups was significant, the SI was compared with and without phase normalization, as well as separately for the trunk and lower extremity muscles, to compare the difference between muscle groups. The SI values computed for the trunk muscles only (0.965 ± 0.034 for the control and 0.86 ± 0.10 for the stroke group) showed a difference (**Figure 4B**). However, the SI from the lower limb muscles (0.968 ± 0.026 for the control and 0.9533 ± 0.054 for the stroke group) did not show a difference between the two groups (**Figure 4C**). Therefore, the trunk muscles appear to be the major contributor to the SI difference evident between the two groups.

Due to the discrepancy of the stance-to-swing ratio between groups, the SI from the transition phase of the gait cycle between stance to swing (50-60%) had higher variability than at any other point in the cycle (**Figure 4A**). To eliminate this discrepancy, stance and swing phase timing was normalized to a ratio of 60:40 percent in the gait cycle, and the SI values were compared. When all muscles were contributing, the SI value of the control group was 0.959 ± 0.028 and 0.892 ± 0.066 for the stroke group. As expected, the SI of the control group did not change after timing normalization since phase timing is quite stable in healthy adults (**Figure 5A** as compared to **Figure 4A**). However, the SI from the post-stroke group had less variance at 50-70% of the gait cycle, and it significantly decreased at 40% and 90% of the gait cycle in comparison to the control group.

The contribution of the trunk muscles (**Figure 5B**) to the SI difference between groups was significant as compared to the lower limb muscles (**Figure 5C**). The SI of the trunk muscles during the entire gait cycle was 0.969 ± 0.029 for the control group and 0.871 ± 0.104 for the stroke group. The high variability of the SI from the stroke group was observed during the middle of the swing (85-90%) and stance (40%) phases. After phase normalization, SI values at the transition phase (50-75%) from stance to swing increased by 7% while variability decreased by 39% (**Figure 5B**). This variability, caused by a discrepancy in the swing-stance phase, would have increased by 64% if phase normalization had not been applied. The SI value from the lower extremity muscles did not demonstrate any difference between the two groups (0.970 ± 0.026 for control and 0.958 ± 0.038 for stroke). Therefore, phase normalization did

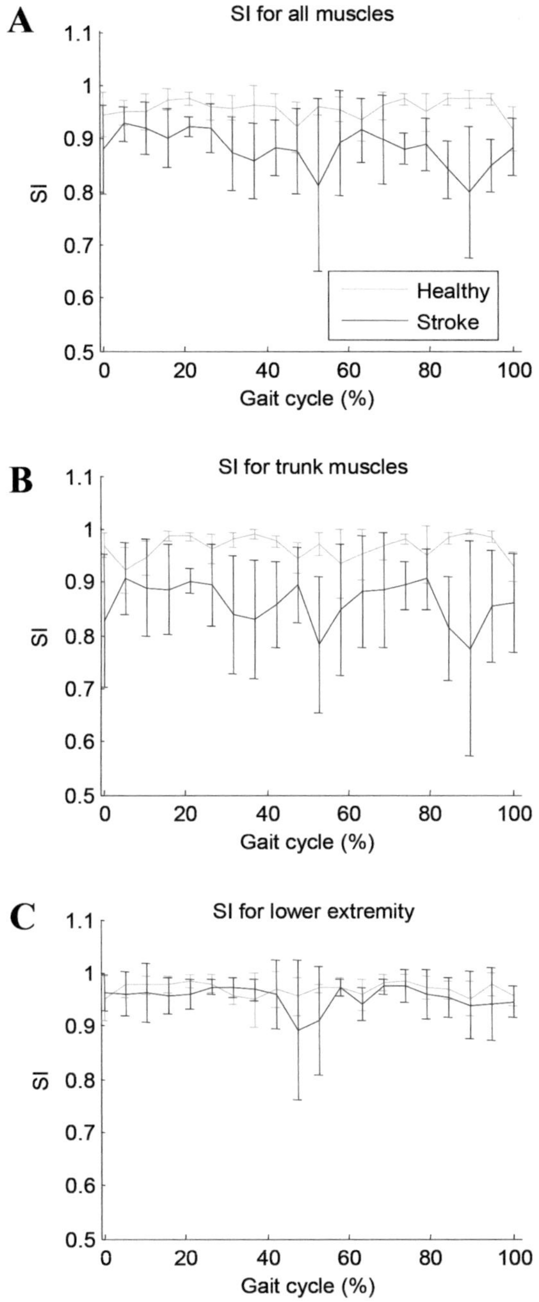

Figure 4.
The SI between control (gray line) and stroke (solid line) groups without phase normalization. The data reveal comparisons between all muscles of the stroke group and the control group (A). The SI comparing back (B) and lower limb muscles (C) indicated that the stroke group revealed increased variability. Although the individual stride EMG from the control group demonstrated consistent patterns with small variability, the stroke group demonstrated larger variability than the control group.

not change any trends seen in the non-timing, normalized SI during the gait cycle, except that the SI variability of the lower extremity muscles (**Figure 5C**) significantly decreased by 50-60% of the gait cycle.

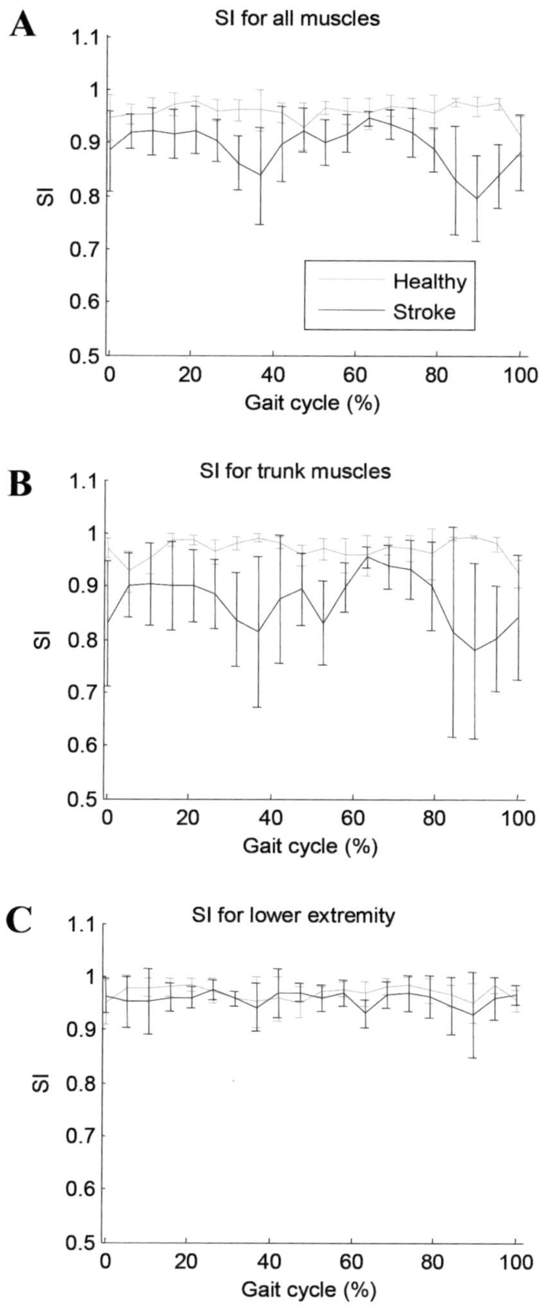

Figure 5.
The SI between control and stroke groups with phase normalization. The prototype, or control group, SI value was close to 1 with less variance in the healthy group than the post-stroke group (A). The data from trunk (B) and lower limb muscles (C) indicated that the stroke group revealed an increased SI value during the transition from stance to swing. Overall, the SI value from the stroke group had less variance at 50-70% of the gait cycle, and it significantly decreased at 40% and 90% of the gait cycle compared to the control group.

Therefore, these results indicated that phase normalization improves the capability to identify the variability between post-stroke subjects and control subjects. A loss of trunk control during walking may result from a reduction in the strength of trunk musculature, especially on the paretic side. It has been suggested that deficits in muscle strength result in reduced mobility of the pelvis in subjects with hemiparesis, which may be a protective strategy to avoid loss of balance. Individuals post-stroke also demonstrate a slower gait velocity with accompanying residual spatial and temporal trunk asymmetry when compared with the gait in healthy adults. Although the most important factors affecting gait velocity and asymmetry remain unknown, lower limb weakness is an important contributing factor. Therefore, trunk muscle activity needs to be carefully evaluated in post-stroke individuals in static and dynamic positions, in addition to trunk muscle activation patterns during gait performance.

However, one of the clinical problems in using EMG analysis with post-stroke patients is the difficulty in obtaining a valid maximum voluntary contraction, which is one accepted method for normalizing the magnitude of a muscle contraction. Nevertheless, previous research examining EMG post-stroke has assessed not only the gait cycle timing of muscle contraction through duration-referenced normalization [45], but also the relative magnitude of muscle contractions for individual muscle groups using some variation of mean or peak activity-referenced norms.

The SI is a reliable measurement of voluntary motor control for move-and-hold tasks [27]; however, the SI has not been used during gait analysis. In this study, timing normalization for phases of gait was necessary post-stroke due to timing variability (see **Figure 4** without normalization as compared to **Figure 5** with timing normalization) found in our participants. In normalizing EMG amplitude, several approaches were available for examining gait post-stroke. In gait analysis, however, peak and mean normalization are commonly accepted ways of examining the relative magnitude of muscle activity. According to the analysis by Benoit and colleagues [44], the peak EMG value is better able to identify pathological groups than average values.

The normalized EMG reflects both the timing of muscle activation and deactivation as well as the relative EMG amplitude of muscle activities. Although the SI itself does not depict the direction of variance from normal muscle activity, the amplitude of normalized EMG data shows the relative muscle activation and deactivation during the gait cycle. Originally, the SI was developed from a move-and-hold task. In addition, the SI has been used with neurologically impaired individuals as well as healthy adults [27, 29, 30]. The SI offers an important contribution to the development of evidence-based treatment evaluation in that the values produced are entirely objective. Therefore, the feasibility of using the SI to quantify the dynamic motor task of gait EMG post-stroke was explored in this study.

4. Summary of gait assessment by the SI

We examined the utilization of the SI as a sensitive tool for the conditions of musculoskeletal and neurologic dysfunctions. Individuals with neck pain have impairments of posture, balance, and coordination as well as sensorimotor deficits. The kinematic SI during gait was useful for clinical outcome measures to differentiate kinematic changes and to demonstrate quantified similarities in the gait cycle between subjects with and without neck pain. These compensatory motions are reflected by altered coordination and muscular control during the gait cycle.

The results of our EMG study in the post-stroke group indicated abnormalities in trunk muscle activity during both the swing and stance phases of gait, especially between the post-stroke and control groups. Although not completed as part of this analysis, the SI could be utilized to examine the differences, if any, in the anterior versus posterior trunk muscles bilaterally as well as hemiparetic to non-hemiparetic responses. The EMG patterns of the post-stroke and control groups during the gait cycle were analyzed by the SI, which computes the similarity of spatial and temporal distributions of muscle activity against the patterns from a control group.

A similar concept could be utilized between pathological and normal responses, as older adults with musculoskeletal dysfunction often have poor neuromuscular control, which may alter normal postural stability. Thus, there is a need to identify specific gait deviations to maintain balance and to develop effective, evidence-based strategies to improve balance control in individuals with balance deficits and to reduce their risk of falls. More importantly, the SI was a sensitive tool used to quantify the characteristics of EMG patterns when proper muscles were selected in subjects with neuromuscular dysfunction. Consequently, the compensatory limb motions resulted in increased motion variabilities and reduced smoothness of limb motions in the gait cycle. Therefore, the development and use of SI may provide an effective means to quantify muscle activity during gait. This, in turn, will assist in establishing effective treatment strategies for gait impairments as well as provide clinical insights into neuromuscular timing abnormalities, specifically for trunk musculature. The SI measure needs to be utilized to analyze gait dysfunction and rehabilitation strategies.

Author details

Paul S. Sung[1*] and Dongchul Lee[2]

1 Department of Physical Therapy, Indiana Wesleyan University, Marion, IN, United States

2 Nevro Inc., Redwood City, California, USA

*Address all correspondence to: drpsung@gmail.com

References

[1] Shaffer SW, Harrison AL. Aging of the somatosensory system: a translational perspective. Physical Therapy. 2007;**87**:193-207

[2] Qiu F, Cole MH, Davids KW, Hennig EM, Silburn PA, Netscher H, et al. Enhanced somatosensory information decreases postural sway in older people. Gait & Posture. 2012;**35**:630-635

[3] Towne SD Jr, Ory MG, Smith ML. Cost of fall-related hospitalizations among older adults: environmental comparisons from the 2011 Texas hospital inpatient discharge data. Population Health Management. 2014;**17**:351-356

[4] Deger TB, Sarac ZF, Savas ES, Akcicek SF. The Relationship of Balance Disorders with Falling, the Effect of Health Problems, and Social Life on Postural Balance in the Elderly Living in a District in Turkey. Geriatrics (Basel). 2019;**4**:37

[5] Schlenstedt C, Brombacher S, Hartwigsen G, Weisser B, Moller B, Deuschl G. Comparison of the Fullerton Advanced Balance Scale, Mini-BESTest, and Berg Balance Scale to Predict Falls in Parkinson Disease. Physical Therapy. 2016;**96**:494-501

[6] Herman T, Inbar-Borovsky N, Brozgol M, Giladi N, Hausdorff JM. The Dynamic Gait Index in healthy older adults: the role of stair climbing, fear of falling and gender. Gait & Posture. 2009;**29**:237-241

[7] Sung PS. Different coordination and flexibility of the spine and pelvis during lateral bending between young and older adults. Human Movement Science. 2016;**46**:229-238

[8] Sung PS, Danial P. Gender difference of shoulder-pelvic kinematic integration for trunk rotation directions in healthy older adults. Clinical Biomechanics (Bristol, Avon). 2017;**50**:56-62

[9] Sung PS. Increased double limb support times during walking in right limb dominant healthy older adults with low bone density. Gait & Posture. 2018;**63**:145-149

[10] Horak FB. Postural orientation and equilibrium: what do we need to know about neural control of balance to prevent falls? Age and Ageing. 2006;**35**(Suppl. 2):ii7-ii11

[11] Horak FB, Wrisley DM, Frank J. The balance evaluation systems test (BESTest) to differentiate balance deficits. Physical Therapy. 2009;**89**:484

[12] Mancini M, Horak FB. The relevance of clinical balance assessment tools to differentiate balance deficits. European Journal of Physical and Rehabilitation Medicine. 2010;**46**:239-248

[13] Patil NS, Dingwell JB, Cusumano JP. Task-level regulation enhances global stability of the simplest dynamic walker. J R Soc Interface. 2020;**17**:20200278

[14] Cusumano JP, Cesari P. Body-goal variability mapping in an aiming task. Biological Cybernetics. 2006;**94**:367-379

[15] Papa EV, Dong X, Hassan M. Resistance training for activity limitations in older adults with skeletal muscle function deficits: a systematic review. Clinical Interventions in Aging. 2017;**12**:955-961

[16] Martin KL, Blizzard L, Wood AG, Srikanth V, Thomson R, Sanders LM,

et al. Cognitive function, gait, and gait variability in older people: a population-based study. The journals of gerontology Series A, Biological sciences and medical sciences. 2013;**68**:726-732

[17] Callisaya ML, Blizzard L, Schmidt MD, Martin KL, McGinley JL, Sanders LM, et al. Gait, gait variability and the risk of multiple incident falls in older people: a population-based study. Age and Ageing. 2011;**40**:481-487

[18] Ferrari R, Russell AS. Regional musculoskeletal conditions: neck pain. Best Practice & Research. Clinical Rheumatology. 2003;**17**:57-70

[19] Cohen SP. Epidemiology, diagnosis, and treatment of neck pain. Mayo Clinic Proceedings. 2015;**90**:284-299

[20] Silva AG, Cruz AL. Standing balance in patients with whiplash-associated neck pain and idiopathic neck pain when compared with asymptomatic participants: A systematic review. Physiotherapy Theory and Practice. 2013;**29**:1-18

[21] Treleaven J. Sensorimotor disturbances in neck disorders affecting postural stability, head and eye movement control. Manual Therapy. 2008;**13**:2-11

[22] Jorgensen MB, Skotte JH, Holtermann A, Sjogaard G, Petersen NC, Sogaard K. Neck pain and postural balance among workers with high postural demands - a cross-sectional study. BMC Musculoskeletal Disorders. 2011;**12**:176

[23] Lee D, Sung PS. Comparison of kinematic similarity index during gait between adults with and without nonspecific chronic neck pain. Gait & Posture. 2022;**91**:99-104

[24] Kirmizi M, Simsek IE, Elvan A, Akcali O, Angin S. Gait speed and gait asymmetry in individuals with chronic idiopathic neck pain. Musculoskeletal Science & Practice. 2019;**41**:23-27

[25] Kadaba MP, Ramakrishnan HK, Wootten ME. Measurement of lower extremity kinematics during level walking. Journal of Orthopaedic Research. 1990;**8**:383-392

[26] Boudarham J, Roche N, Pradon D, Bonnyaud C, Bensmail D, Zory R. Variations in kinematics during clinical gait analysis in stroke patients. PLoS One. 2013;**8**:e66421

[27] Lee DC, Lim HK, McKay WB, Priebe MM, Holmes SA, Sherwood AM. Toward an objective interpretation of surface EMG patterns: a voluntary response index (VRI). Journal of Electromyography and Kinesiology. 2004;**14**:379-388

[28] Lim HK, Lee DC, McKay WB, Priebe MM, Holmes SA, Sherwood AM. Neurophysiological assessment of lower-limb voluntary control in incomplete spinal cord injury. Spinal Cord. 2005;**43**:283-290

[29] Lim HK, Lee DC, McKay WB, Protas EJ, Holmes SA, Priebe MM, et al. Analysis of sEMG during voluntary movement--Part II: Voluntary response index sensitivity. IEEE Transactions on Neural Systems and Rehabilitation Engineering. 2004;**12**:416-421

[30] McKay WB, Lee DC, Lim HK, Holmes SA, Sherwood AM. Neurophysiological examination of the corticospinal system and voluntary motor control in motor-incomplete human spinal cord injury. Experimental Brain Research. 2005;**163**:379-387

[31] McKay WB, Lim HK, Priebe MM, Stokic DS, Sherwood AM. Clinical neurophysiological assessment of

residual motor control in post-spinal cord injury paralysis. Neurorehabilitation and Neural Repair. 2004;**18**:144-153

[32] Sung PS, Danial P. A Kinematic Symmetry Index of Gait Patterns Between Older Adults With and Without Low Back Pain. Spine (Phila Pa). 1976;**2017**(42):E1350-E13E6

[33] Alsultan F, De Nunzio AM, Rushton A, Heneghan NR, Falla D. Variability of neck and trunk movement during single- and dual-task gait in people with chronic neck pain. Clinical Biomechanics (Bristol, Avon). 2020;**72**:31-36

[34] Falla D, Gizzi L, Parsa H, Dieterich A, Petzke F. People With Chronic Neck Pain Walk With a Stiffer Spine. The Journal of Orthopaedic and Sports Physical Therapy. 2017;**47**:268-277

[35] Sung PS, Danial P, Lee DC. Reliability of the Kinematic Steadiness Index during one-leg standing in subjects with recurrent low back pain. European Spine Journal. 2018;**27**:171-179

[36] Stanton TR, Leake HB, Chalmers KJ, Moseley GL. Evidence of Impaired Proprioception in Chronic, Idiopathic Neck Pain: Systematic Review and Meta-Analysis. Physical Therapy. 2016;**96**:876-887

[37] Perry J. Gait Analysis: Normal and Pathological Function. Thorofare, NJ: SLACK Inc.; 1992

[38] Woodhouse A, Vasseljen O. Altered motor control patterns in whiplash and chronic neck pain. BMC Musculoskeletal Disorders. 2008;**9**:90

[39] Huang YP, Bruijn SM, Lin JH, Meijer OG, Wu WH, Abbasi-Bafghi H, et al. Gait adaptations in low back pain patients with lumbar disc herniation: trunk coordination and arm swing. European Spine Journal. 2011;**20**:491-499

[40] van Dieen JH, Prins MR, Bruijn SM, Wu WH, Liang B, Lamoth CJC, et al. Coordination of Axial Trunk Rotations During Gait in Low Back Pain. A Narrative Review. J Hum Kinet. 2021;**76**:35-50

[41] Van Criekinge T, Saeys W, Hallemans A, Velghe S, Viskens PJ, Vereeck L, et al. Trunk biomechanics during hemiplegic gait after stroke: A systematic review. Gait & Posture. 2017;**54**:133-143

[42] Lodha N, Chen YT, McGuirk TE, Fox EJ, Kautz SA, Christou EA, et al. EMG synchrony to assess impaired corticomotor control of locomotion after stroke. Journal of Electromyography and Kinesiology. 2017;**37**:35-40

[43] Van Criekinge T, Truijen S, Schroder J, Maebe Z, Blanckaert K, van der Waal C, et al. The effectiveness of trunk training on trunk control, sitting and standing balance and mobility post-stroke: a systematic review and meta-analysis. Clinical Rehabilitation. 2019;**33**:992-1002

[44] Benoit D, Lamontagne M, Cerulli G, Liti A. The clinical significance of electromyography normalisation techniques in subjects with anterior cruciate ligament injury during treadmill walking. Gait and Posture. 2003;**18**:56-63

[45] Knutson L, Soderberg G. EMG: Use and Interpretation in Gait. In: Craig RL, Oatis CA, editors. Gait Analysis: Theory & Applications. St. Louis: Mosby; 1995. pp. 307-325